Access your online resources

The Speech and Language Activity Resource Book is accompanied by a number of printable online materials designed to ensure this resource best supports your professional needs.

Activate your online resources:

Go to www.routledge.com/cw/speechmark and click on the cover of this book.

Click the 'Sign in or Request Access' button and follow the instructions in order to access the resources.

The Speech and Language Activity Resource Book

The Speech and Language Activity Resource Book offers a flexible and readily available set of activities and worksheets designed to support speech and language therapists as they deliver personalised and engaging therapy sessions.

With topics based on seasons, hobbies, sports and celebrations, etc, the worksheets can be selected to suit a client's interests as well as targeting specific skills and needs. The engaging activities encourage conversation and participation, promoting skill development in a way that is easily translated into everyday communication.

Key features of this book include:

- A range of activities, arranged by level of difficulty, that can be selected based on the client's individual need
- A person-centred approach to therapy, enabling the time-poor practitioner the opportunity to personalise their care with ease
- Photocopiable and downloadable sheets that can be completed during therapy sessions or sent out to the client for home practice, as well as blank worksheets that can be used to create new, appropriate activities

Easily adaptable for group sessions, one-on-one therapy sessions and home activities, this is an essential tool for speech and language therapists and occupational therapists, as well as families and other practitioners supporting adults with a range of acquired communication difficulties.

Tracy Broadley Jackson has over 30 years of experience as a speech and language therapist, developing her skills across a variety of clinical settings. She has worked with a range of clients throughout her career, including people with voice and fluency difficulties and those with communication problems arising from acute brain damage and neurodegenerative conditions such as Parkinson's and dementia.

Currently, she has two roles. Firstly, as an independent speech and language therapist, running her own practice, Speakmore. Secondly, she works for the NHS in a mental health hospital as part of a multidisciplinary team across in-patient wards.

Delivering person-centred care is at the heart of her work; knowing a client's interests and hobbies is key to helping that person remain motivated and express themselves in a way that allows them to be the unique individual they are. This approach inspired her to produce *The Speech and Language Activity Resource Book* and share with colleagues the activities that have shaped her individual and group therapy sessions.

THE SPEECH AND LANGUAGE ACTIVITY RESOURCE BOOK

THEMED THERAPY SESSIONS FOR ADULTS

TRACY BROADLEY JACKSON

Routledge
Taylor & Francis Group
LONDON AND NEW YORK

First published 2022
by Routledge
4 Park Square, Milton Park, Abingdon, Oxon OX14 4RN

and by Routledge
605 Third Avenue, New York, NY 10158

Routledge is an imprint of the Taylor & Francis Group, an informa business

British Library Cataloguing-in-Publication Data
A catalogue record for this book is available from the British Library

Library of Congress Cataloging-in-Publication Data
Names: Broadley Jackson, Tracy, author.
Title: The speech and language activity resource book : themed therapy sessions for adults/Tracy Broadley Jackson.
Description: Milton Park, Abingdon, Oxon; New York, NY: Routledge, 2022. |
Includes bibliographical references and index.
Identifiers: LCCN 2021036352 (print) | LCCN 2021036353 (ebook) |
ISBN 9781032012452 (hardback) | ISBN 9781032012445 (paperback) |
ISBN 9781003177852 (ebook)
Subjects: LCSH: Speech therapy.
Classification: LCC RC423 .B735 2022 (print) | LCC RC423 (ebook) |
DDC 616.85/506–dc23
LC record available at https://lccn.loc.gov/2021036352
LC ebook record available at https://lccn.loc.gov/2021036353

ISBN: 978-1-032-01245-2 (hbk)
ISBN: 978-1-032-01244-5 (pbk)
ISBN: 978-1-003-17785-2 (ebk)

DOI: 10.4324/9781003177852

Typeset in Univers
by Deanta Global Publishing Services, Chennai, India

Access the companion website: www.routledge.com/cw/speechmark

For Product Safety Concerns and Information please contact our EU representative:
GPSR@taylorandfrancis.com
Taylor & Francis Verlag GmbH, Kaufingerstraße 24, 80331 München, Germany

CONTENTS

ACKNOWLEDGEMENTS

This book has been a labour of love, but I could not have completed it without the help and support of my wonderful family and friends.

My first thanks go to Debra Mann, who inspired me to consider developing themed therapy sessions. This advice has had a profound impact on the way I deliver therapy.

Thank you to Kate Jackson, who assisted with the first chapter and really got me started. My gratitude, too, for your ongoing support, advice and faith in me.

Thank you to Sam Jackson for providing endless enthusiasm and checking I was alright throughout my writings. Your energy always inspires me.

Numerous friends read various drafts of the resource, providing invaluable feedback and encouragement, including Clare Mason, Tracey Skeet, Jackie Dornford-May, Kim Edwards, Fiona and Graham Blagg.

I am very grateful to Neil Bonner and Darren Kinnersley-Hill, who so kindly allowed me to use their excellent limericks – thank you.

I am indebted to my numerous colleagues and students who, throughout my working life, have passed on tips and ideas for delivering client-centred therapy.

Thank you to my clients and their families who have inspired me to keep my therapy sessions somewhere they can laugh, relax and enjoy interacting.

I am grateful to the team at Routledge and Speechmark publishing for their support, guidance and patience.

Last but not least, a huge thank you goes to my husband Dave, who has patiently worked away in the background to keep me fed, the house and dog running, and enabled me to concentrate on this book.

INTRODUCTION

Aim of the book

This book aims to provide a wide range of activities to be used by anybody promoting communication and engagement in adults with or without communication difficulties. It has been compiled following years of delivering themed therapy sessions for clients. In my experience, this approach generates natural conversation, maintains motivation and provides cohesion to the sessions. I am passionate about offering therapy in this manner and would love you to be inspired by the themes and activities in this resource.

The book is arranged into 20 themed chapters to cater for a range of interests. As therapists, clients and carers, we invest a lot of time in therapy, which should be fun, interesting and meaningful, rather than a set of exercises using random topics. The evidence indicates that when therapy is geared towards the person's interests and is relevant to their everyday communication, they will be more motivated and make better progress (Bruce & Newton, 2018; Ramig & Fox, 2008). For the busy clinician, it can be time-consuming to develop relevant and varied resources for clients.

Therapists should seek to discover the person behind the communication difficulty, encompassing a social rather than solely an individual or medical model (Jordan & Bryan, 2001; Cooney & O'Shea, 2018). Using relevant therapy topics reinforces and supports this approach (Kitwood, 2011). To learn more about the person, therapists could use the 'About Me' questionnaire in Appendix 2 to elicit information about their life and interests.

The vocabulary within the activities has been chosen to elicit responses using a range of word classes. Although the topics are specific, most of the vocabulary chosen is intended to reflect everyday words.

The activities are designed to be utilised with a range of different verbal and written communication difficulties and situations, including:

1. communication difficulties (speech, language, voice, fluency)
2. causes of the problem (e.g. stroke, dementia, Parkinson's)
3. facilitators (e.g. speech and language therapist, occupational therapist, activity coordinator, psychologist, family member, friend)
4. settings (e.g. own home, hospital, day centre, community centre)
5. methods of delivery, i.e. one-to-one or group.

Who can use this resource?

a) The worksheets will be used by speech and language therapists to support carefully designed, targeted therapy programmes. Delivering therapy exercises that are interesting and meaningful is an essential component in motivating clients. As busy clinicians, it is always great to have professional-looking, ready-made worksheets to hand.

b) Many of the activities in this book will be useful for other healthcare workers such as activity coordinators, occupational therapists, psychologists and nurses, all of whom could potentially run groups for people requiring interaction and cognitive-language stimulation.

c) It is also intended for people living with a communication difficulty to use independently with or without the help of a family member, friend, or carer to supplement work provided by a speech and language therapist. Furthermore, the activities could offer the family and friends of a person with a communication difficulty a means to interact and connect in a way that is more difficult in day-to-day interactions.

What is a communication difficulty?

It is estimated that 20 per cent of the adult population will experience a communication disorder at some point in their life. For example, a third of stroke survivors will experience some degree of communication difficulty (RCSLT). There are many reasons why communication might be impaired and can range from being a life-long problem to a new one with the onset of a condition such as dementia, Parkinson's or traumatic brain damage.

Difficulties in communicating can arise when somebody struggles to express themselves in spoken words and in writing. Other people have difficulty understanding what is being said to them, or being able to read.[1] Some people struggle with several aspects of communication. The difficulties targeted in this resource are classified into four basic categories: (i) speech; (ii) language, (iii) problems using voice correctly and (iv) fluency. See the chapter, 'How to use this resource', Table 1, for more information about speech, language, voice and fluency.

While speech and language therapists play a vital role in assessing, diagnosing and treating communication difficulties, they do not carry sole responsibility for facilitating enhanced communication in people with communication difficulties. Speech and language therapists provide specialist treatment, but everybody can contribute to enabling each individual to interact and engage at some level.

Why is communication so important?

> *Conversation is the essence of human interaction and the cement of human relationships. It is the window on to thought, and its flow is what most of us take for granted in all our everyday encounters.*
>
> *(Claire Penn, 2001)*[2]

Communication is a sophisticated and complex process that separates us from other animals. It involves many parts of the brain to process the words and formulate a response. It allows us to share and obtain thoughts, feelings and information. It enables us to build and maintain relationships. Unfortunately, it is a skill that can be lost or difficult to maintain when changes to the brain occur as a result of a disease or accident. Anybody talking to somebody with a communication difficulty will be aware of the difficulties, constraints and communication breakdown that can occur when the process is interrupted by a condition such as a voice loss or slurred speech in dysarthria. The importance of enabling people to communicate and engage with others cannot be overstated. The impact of communication difficulties on people's mental health is well documented across the range of disorders including aphasia (Währborg, 1991; Hilari & Northcott, 2017), dysarthria (Walshe & Miller, 2011), dysphonia (voice loss) (Misono et al., 2016 Andrea et al., 2018) and dysfluency (Yaruss, 2010; Lucey et al., 2019). The NICE guideline NG97 for people with dementia, clearly summarises this impact, stating that 'difficulties interacting with other people can cause psychological symptoms such as depressed mood, which can then make the difficulties worse, causing a cycle'.

As well as providing a resource for therapists working with people with communication disorders, this resource aims to provide material which bridges the gap of communication difficulties by advocating activities to facilitate interaction.

Notes

1 Communication is a complex process and the description provided does not reflect this. However, the definition given here is for the purpose of this resource and the difficulties it helps to address.

2 Quote in the resource by Lock et al., 2008.

HOW TO USE THIS RESOURCE

This resource was developed to provide a series of enjoyable, interesting, and easy access worksheets for adults with communication difficulties. This chapter explains in more detail how to implement the activities whether you are a speech and language therapist, other healthcare provider, a family member, a friend or the person with a communication difficulty. This resource is not a therapy programme, and if in doubt, you are advised to seek the advice of a qualified speech and language therapist.

It is anticipated that whoever delves into this book will have different skills and experiences of communication difficulties. Speech and language therapists are very skilled and experienced in diagnosing and treating communication disorders. They are knowledgeable about therapy strategies to facilitate the client's communication. I hope this resource will be an inspiration and adjunct to their existing material. In contrast, some people looking at this book might know less or be new to the arena of communication difficulties; it has also been written with this in mind. Therefore, whilst it is not a substitute for a comprehensive speech and language assessment and intervention plan, it is designed for non-speech and language therapists to use. The information below is intended to inform both speech and language therapists and non-speech and language therapists how to use the book.

The book consists of 20 themed chapters, each containing various activities; an appendix of blank activity templates; and an 'About Me' questionnaire. Every activity has a difficulty rating, called a 'level'. There are three difficulty levels, and they are described in Section 2 of this chapter. To help the reader navigate the resource, a table of contents is given at the beginning of each chapter detailing:

- ❑ activity and page number
- ❑ activity description (e.g. anagram, word search and so on)
- ❑ which client group the activity is most suited to (i.e. speech, voice, language, fluency or any of these in a group setting)
- ❑ activity difficulty level
- ❑ suggestions about how the activity might be modified or used. For example, how to make it easier, more challenging, or identifying that it would work particularly well as a group activity.

At the end of each chapter is a 'words of increasing length' activity. This list is not referenced in the contents page for each theme as it appears at the end of every chapter.

The blank activity templates in Appendix 1 are primarily designed for speech and language therapists to enable them to expand the range of activities for topics covered in the book. Additionally, it is anticipated that they could be used to create activities for clients with interests not covered in this resource. The templates could also be used by anybody who feels confident enough to develop activities for their clients or family member.

Appendix 2 is a questionnaire for the client or their significant person to complete. The information will enable the therapist to incorporate the client's interests into the sessions, ensuring therapy is meaningful and motivating.

The remainder of this chapter provides the following information:

1) A list of definitions for some words used in this book.
2) An explanation of the different levels of difficulty.
3) How to use this resource as a speech and language therapist.
4) How to use this resource as a non-speech and language therapist (including recommendations on how to elicit the best response from the person).
5) Modifying the activities: ideas about how to adjust the activities to make them harder, easier or develop the task into further exercises.
6) How to use the word lists (words of increasing length activities at the end of each chapter).
7) General information.

1. Definitions

See Table 1 on the next page.

2. Difficulty levels

The chapters are not arranged into a hierarchical sequence of activities from easy to hard. However, some individual activities are designed to be graded with increasing levels of challenge. When this occurs, the activity is given a letter: a, b, c and so on. Letter (a) is usually the easiest, with difficulty increasing on subsequent letters.

For example, in Chapter 3 (Autumn), Activity 2, a word search, starts as '2(a)' words provided; '2(b)' pictures and anagrams; and '2(c)' pictures only (which is harder as the person has to recall the word and spell it before finding it in the word search).

Table 1 Definitions of words used throughout this resource

TERM	MEANING
Activity	The activity is the task described on each page. The activity is also referred to as 'task' or 'exercise'.
Additional activity ideas	At the bottom of some activities, additional ideas are provided to help elicit more communication from the client.
Client	The client is the person with communication difficulties who is being helped or is helping themself – also called 'the person'.
Client Group	Communication difficulties are categorised into different types of disorders depending on which part of communicating is a problem: speech, language, voice, fluency. See below for further information.
Fluency	The rhythm, timing and flow of speech.
Instructions	At the top of each worksheet, there are instructions on how to complete the activity.
Language	Using words, putting words into sentences, reading, writing and understanding the words spoken by others.
Levels	The difficulty level of each activity is labelled 1, 2 or 3. See Table 2 for more information.
Speech	The sounds we produce with our tongue, lips and teeth; articulation.
The person	'The person' refers to the individual with a communication difficulty. Also referred to as 'the client' or 'the individual' in other parts of the book.
Theme	Also referred to as the 'topic' in the book. This refers to the theme within the chapter, such as 'films', 'birds' or 'summer' and so on.
Therapist	Usually refers to Speech and Language Therapist, but might also be Occupational Therapist, activity Coordinator or Psychologist.
Voice	Voice is the sound produced by the voice box (larynx).

Each activity is given a rating of easy (suitable for Level 1), medium (suitable for Level 2) or hard (suitable for Level 3). See Table 2 on the next page for more information. The levels reflect the person's ability to express themselves, read, write or understand what others say to them. Communication is much more complicated than this might suggest, but it guides the most appropriate activity for an individual within the chapter.

The levels do not account for how well a person interacts with others or participates in conversations or how confident they might feel communicating. However, it might be helpful to consider these aspects when selecting an activity.

The levels are for guidance only, so when choosing an activity, check the task first to decide whether you or your client can manage it. An activity should provide some challenge but not be so hard that no parts of it are achievable. Be prepared to choose a more straightforward activity if the one being practised is not enjoyable or attainable.

Table 2 Client levels

LEVEL	ABBREVIATION	EXPLANATION	EXAMPLES
Level 1	L1	The person has significant difficulty with speech, voice, language or fluency. They might need a lot of help to achieve the task or encouragement to complete it.	Severe difficulty recalling everyday words after a stroke.
Level 2	L2	The person can communicate reasonably well but frequently stops or adjusts their message to compensate for their difficulty.	Conveys most of their message but has frequent hesitations, errors and may struggle to use whole sentences, e.g. somebody with dementia.
Level 3	L3	The person may not present as having a difficulty initially but struggles in certain situations such as groups.	Somebody with a mild voice or fluency difficulty.

3. How to use this resource – speech and language therapists

a) Choosing a task

In this section, some ideas are offered about how to use the tasks with particular client groups. Clinicians must utilise their knowledge and experience alongside client feedback to establish a relevant intervention programme with appropriate activities to support that plan.

- ❑ The resource has been produced to provide material for use during therapy sessions and home practice. At the bottom of the activity pages, a heading – '**Therapy Targets**' – is provided for the therapist to add specific notes and prompts for the skill the client is focusing on. For example, you might prompt the client to 'use full sentences', or 'exaggerate your speech', depending on the target. Alternatively, use this space to indicate how often they should practise each day. In this way, the task is personalised to your client's goals.

- ❑ As a speech and language therapist, you will be familiar with the WHO classification of Functioning, Disability and Health (ICF). Based on your assessment findings, hypothesis about the nature of the problem and your client's goals, you will identify which interventions to target in terms of impairment, activity, or participation. Some activities, such as single word recall tasks, naturally lend themselves to working at an impairment-based level, particularly aphasia and apraxia. Some worksheets promote practise at the level of 'activity', e.g. Activity 3 in Chapter 13, which could be used as a prompt for writing a shopping list. Others exercises form the structure for practising a specific technique or strategy. As speech and language therapists, we are skilled at helping clients practise strategies known to improve speech intelligibility in dysarthria (Enderby, 2013) or voice techniques in dysphonia (Martin & Lockhart, 2013); there are plenty of activities in the resource for this purpose. Exercises such as sentence reading, prose and poetry are ideal starting points to embed the strategy into everyday speech. To facilitate participation, therapists should choose activities such as games and discussion topics.

- When selecting a task, therapists need to acknowledge that, depending upon the goal, there might be cross-over of impairment, disability or participation and that working on one aspect might influence another. This principle is illustrated in the study by Herbert et al. (2003), who used conversation analysis to identify whether working at the impairment level improved conversation in people with aphasia. Their results supported a positive impact on conversation (participation) via impairment-based therapy. These findings are corroborated in the literature review by Carragher et al. (2012).

- Although the tasks are not set out in a strict hierarchical order, the difficulty levels L1–L3 assist with designing a graded hierarchy of intervention. For example, increasing linguistic demands during speech tasks has been reported to adversely affect fluency in people who stammer (Blombgren & Goberman, 2008). When introducing a strategy, begin with L1 activities, so the emphasis can be solely the strategy, before moving to more demanding tasks. As a case example, consider a 20-year-old student who wants to improve his fluency when talking with friends. He is working on respiratory support to help control the pace of speech output. After practising breath control at rest, he begins practising breath support by reading aloud 'words with increasing length'. When he feels comfortable at this level, the speaking load increases using short, spontaneous speech tasks such as naming objects in a rucksack (Activity 2(c) in Chapter 16), before increasing the challenge to a conversation task, (e.g. in Chapter 16, Activity 5 is designed to stimulate discussion and explanation). Obviously, therapeutic intervention is more complex than implied above, but the example serves to illustrate how the client could build their skills and confidence by working through the different task levels available in this book.

- Challenging clients cognitively whilst practising their communication skills simulates real-life situations. It is well-known that most people struggle to dual-task effectively (Dromey & Shim, 2008), and it becomes even more challenging in certain conditions such as Parkinson's. Typically, word recall, as reflected in verbal fluency, reduces when the individual with Parkinson's carries out another task such as walking or standing (Dromey et al., 2010). Therefore, tasks requiring the person to use different executive functions will challenge their focus on word recall. This has certainly been my experience with this client group. A game such as Activity 1 in Chapter 16, 'I went camping and forgot to take…' incorporates many of these distractions. It has proved to be an enjoyable activity, and when I have used it in groups, has been a great way to encourage gesture as participants mime their item to remind the speaker what they named in their turn.

- Poor breath support and high linguistic demands might impair speech production in some clients, such as those with Parkinson's (Huber & Darling, 2011). Word recall tasks might help increase the person's awareness of such difficulties and enable them to apply strategies to overcome them. A task with lower word recall demands, such as reading a poem aloud, could support both the linguistic abilities as well as the strategies being taught for better breath control and intonation.

- For more information about the hierarchy of tasks in fluency and voice, therapists are guided to review specific literature and resources such as *The Dysfluency Resource Book* by Turnbull and Stewart (2010) and *Working with Voice Disorders* by Martin and Lockhart (2013).

b) Evidence-base

In terms of therapy efficacy, each clinician's responsibility is to consider the evidence base for any techniques used in their interventions. Therapists will devise their treatment plan to take into account each client's needs, strengths and interests. There is a plethora of research investigating therapy effectiveness across the communication difficulty sub-types. When devising a plan, clinicians will be guided by research relevant to their client, their own experiences and the client's response to therapy. The rich complexity of client presentations and the range of therapy techniques are too extensive and complex to reference each activity type used in this resource. Some guiding principles for dysfluency and voice therapy have already been outlined above. A few studies that support using the activities in aphasia and apraxia therapy are discussed briefly below.

- Word retrieval in aphasia, and aphasia with apraxia of speech, benefit from semantic feature analysis treatment (Dominique et al., 2021). Semantic tasks in the resource include ideas-webs, word association and matching tasks. For example, Activity 8 in Chapter 10 could stimulate semantic associations when matching a bird type to a colour.

- The rationale behind the use of anagrams, completing missing letters in words and reading words loud is detailed in *Semantic and Naming Therapy* by Cardell and Lawrie (2013). They outline how targeting specific processes within a cognitive neuropsychological model helps to strengthen word recall.

- In the study by Herbert et al. (2003), facilitating word recall in sentences was shown to have a greater positive impact on conversation in aphasia treatment than single word recall. Many activities in this resource employ single word recall, progressing to sentence production using those target words.

- In the section for family and friends, 'Tips to help with word-finding and spelling', ideas are given regarding the types of cues that might help somebody with aphasia to recall words. They are provided in a non-hierarchical order. Speech and language therapists wishing to explore this area further should review the literature (e.g. Patterson, 2001).

c) Group therapy

- Many activities in this resource are either recommended for or can be adapted for group therapy. Check the contents page of each chapter to find suitable group activities. Client type and group aims will vary, and it might even be appropriate to mix up client sub-types within one group, for example, having somebody with apraxia alongside somebody with dysarthria. This would allow the clinician to focus on the level of functioning or confidence rather than diagnosis when designing a group. The activity level chosen will correlate to the needs of the group. The nature, range and extent of group types is too extensive to review therapy efficacy here, especially with regards to information about specific therapy tasks. Therapists are encouraged to use outcome measures to gauge the effectiveness of the group intervention. In a clinical setting, the measure should reflect meaningful change for the participants. In their review of group therapy for people with dysarthria, Whillans et al. (2020) suggested that group therapy 'may improve speech production and in some cases communicative effectiveness or wellbeing'. Elman et al. (1999) demonstrated long-term benefits in group therapy for people with aphasia. The focus of therapy was initiation of conversation and 'exchanging information using whatever communicative means possible'. Many tasks in this resource encourage interaction using an inclusive communication approach. For example, in Chapter 20, Activity 3, clients who cannot name drinks can be provided with pictures and words of healthy and not so healthy drinks to select in order to complete the task.

- The benefits of group therapy will depend on members' goals and expectations. In *Group Treatment of Neurogenic Communication Disorders* (Elman, 2007), various authors discuss group therapy content and activities for clients with dementia, traumatic brain damage and aphasia. In her chapter on group treatment for people with dementia, Hopper reviews a number of studies. She cites studies which measured conversation 'crossover' (Jo & Boczko, 1998) and topic initiation (Arkin & Mahendra, 2001). In their chapter, Garrett et al. explain how the 'scaffold discourse' group model enables clients to use their individual skills to achieve their goal by completing a transaction, describing a procedure or debating a point. Opportunity to practice these skills can be created using the resources in this book. For example, Activity 8 in Chapter 11, asks the person to arrange sentences into the correct order to explain how to do specific gardening tasks. The games and discussion topics in each chapter are ideal for groups to facilitate conversation skills for a range of clients.

d) Outcome measures

Good practice demands the use of outcome measures in our work as speech and language therapists. Measuring outcomes should be integral to the therapist's intervention programme. Identifying the goal of therapy is key to knowing whether the intervention has been effective and whether it needs to be modified. Outcome measures prompt the clinician to consider the focus of their therapy. For example, Therapy Outcome Measures (Enderby et al., 2015) cover four elements of client functioning – impairment, activity, participation and wellbeing. For example, does the client want to ring a friend (activity) or go to the pub (participation). The choice of exercises will reflect these goals and can be measured against the Therapy Outcome Measures. Similarly, the Goal Attainment Scale (Kirusek & Sherman, 1968; King's College, 2021) might influence the therapist to select a specific therapy topic according to the goal topic. An example could be the client who wishes to return to her gardening club; the therapist uses the activities in Chapter 11 to improve her confidence in talking about things related to gardening.

Additionally, since this resource aims to promote the concept that therapy can be enjoyable, therapists could consider using a 'Session Rating Scale' similar to the one applied after a solution-focused therapy session (Bannink, 2010) to measure how satisfied the client is with their session.

4. How to use this resource – relatives, friends, carers and the person with a communication difficulty

For clarity, from this point onward, relatives and carers will be called 'helper'.

Points to consider:

- ❑ The activities are not a test – provide as much help as required to enable the person to carry out the task (see below for the types of prompts).

- ❑ Keep the sessions fun.
- ❑ It doesn't matter how long it takes the person to complete a task. However, if they are struggling a lot, the task might be too hard. Provide help, move on to another task or leave that activity for another time.
- ❑ Doing a little and often is better than spending hours at a time. For example, 15–20 minutes is sufficient time to practise for one session.
- ❑ If the person wants to try doing the activity on their own, that would be an excellent boost for their independence; if you check how they have done, try not to 'mark' it right or wrong. Instead, gently show them the correct answer if you feel that would be helpful.
- ❑ If they are struggling to complete the task or begin to look tired, try something easier or have a rest. You can always try again tomorrow.
- ❑ Try to end a practice session with a task the person can achieve easily to end on a positive note.

Tips to help with word-finding and spelling

When somebody is struggling to find a word, the following prompts can often elicit the word. Prompts are usually called 'cues' by speech and language therapists. The type of cue that helps the most depends on the type of difficulty. In their book, Cardell and Lawrie (2013) describe these difficulties in more detail and identify which cues could help specific deficits. Your speech and language therapist will recommend which cues to use. Some cues that help are listed below:

i. Provide the first sounds of the word. For example, if the word required is 'Yellow', you could say, 'Ye…'.

ii. Write down the first letter of the word and say it out loud if they are still struggling.

iii. Gesture – mime the action with or without the actual object. Imagine somebody is in the garden and you are in the kitchen. You tap on the window to get their attention; then you make a gesture to ask if they want a cup of tea. Use those sorts of everyday, simple gestures.

iv. Offer two alternative options. For example, in Chapter 10, in the activity identifying a bird colour, you could ask, 'Is it yellow or blue?'. Be aware that many people will usually select the last choice, so vary the order you offer for the target word.

v. With spelling activities, use loose letter tiles from games such as scrabble. Place the required letters on the table so they can be moved around to spell the word. This method might be easier than writing the word.

vi. If the person is struggling, try another strategy to prompt the answer. Remember, the aim is for the person to build their confidence, complete and enjoy the task.

5. Modifying the activities

a) Sentences

- ❑ Sentences in the activities can be modified to make them easier or more challenging. For example, in the sentences in Activity 9 from Chapter 4, the therapist or helper could re-write the sentences but remove different words. Often words in the middle will be hardest to find.

Sentence: The fire is winter's fruit.

Options:

a) The ______ is winter's fruit, or

b) The fire is winter's _____

Either suggest words that could be used or write out or draw some options for the client to choose.

- ❑ Single-word activities can be extended by asking the person to make the word into a sentence. For example, when naming words associated with, for example, 'films', ask the person you are working with to put those words into a sentence.

E.g. words associated with films – ticket, horror, *director* and *actors*.

'This *director* always uses loads of famous *actors* in his films'.

b) Passages

Activities that are based around passages are given specific instructions throughout the book. The passages in the book can be used in many ways to promote communication skills. Some ideas include:

- ❑ Identifying word groups, such as action words, adjectives including colours or conjunctions (joining words such as 'and', 'but').
- ❑ Ask the client to read the passage then summarise it.
- ❑ Ask questions about the passage. The questions could be written in the text or be inferred from the information provided.
- ❑ Reading aloud can be a beneficial exercise when practising specific aspects of speech, voice and fluency. It is often used as a step in the journey towards using that skill in everyday life (as described above).
- ❑ Use the passage to stimulate a discussion – ask what else the person knows about the topic, or do they agree with the points made in the passage? This is a great group activity and in my groups usually generates interesting debates and banter.

c) Poems

Poetry as a vehicle for communication therapy is gaining momentum. Interesting articles include the paper by Fujii and Wan (2014) who explore the use of rhythm in conditions such as autism, aphasia and Parkinson's. In my work, poetry has proved to be an excellent vehicle to promote intonation, explore feelings and generate discussion.

The poems in the resource can be used in different ways, depending on the client's needs. Some ideas for how to use the poetry are listed below:

- ❑ Reading aloud to practise general or specific aspects of speech, voice and fluency. Poetry is perfect for practising intonation and rhythm.
- ❑ Use as a backdrop to introduce a word association activity.
- ❑ The therapist could read the poem, then promote a discussion about it. For example, did the client or group enjoy the poem? How did it make them feel? Have they read a similar poem?
- ❑ Poems could be used to encourage people to write their own poem or piece of prose. High functioning clients love this challenge!
- ❑ Find different categories of words amongst the poems. For example, in the poem, 'I made a little snowman' – how many verbs (action words) can they find? Can the person

find other types of words such as adjectives (describing words, e.g. red, big, loud) or prepositions (words that identify the position of one object in relation to another, e.g. below, next to, behind)?

- Poetry fulfils a multitude of purposes and can offer many benefits in therapy. For example, in one study of clients with multiple sclerosis, (Balchin et al., 2020), poetry was found to improve participants' communication confidence.

d) Word searches

Here are some ideas to make the task easier or harder or develop its use.

- To make the task easier, highlight the first letter or two.
- Ask the person to list five other words related to the topic.
- Are there any other words to be found in the word search? Other words may or may not be related to the theme.
- Ask your client to make a sentence with each of the words they find.
- How many of the words can they use in one sentence?
- Ask your client to define the words they find.
- How many words can they find without having any word clues to prompt them.
- Can they make a word search for you to do!

6. Word lists

At the end of each chapter, there is a list of words that increase in length. Each row begins with a one-syllable word; next, there's a two-syllable word followed by two words or a phrase consisting of three or more syllables. Finally, the client is prompted to create a sentence using the longer word or phrase presented in the final column.

For example: Table 3

At the end of each word list there are two blank rows for therapists or clients to insert their own words and phrases.

Table 3 Example of concluding table: words of increasing length

One syllable	Two syllables	Multisyllabic	Now say a complete sentence using the multisyllabic word or phrase
Wrap	Wrapping	Wrapping paper	*"The wrapping paper was shiny."*

7. General information

- Most activities are designed so that answers can be either written or spoken. For example, although word searches are primarily a silent reading exercise, the client could be asked to read aloud the words they have found. Some activities do not lend themselves to being spoken aloud.

- There might be several options for the 'correct' answer. Discussing a client's response is a great way to promote discussion and enhance specific skills such as problem-solving.

- For some activities where the answers might be less readily known or obvious, an answer page is provided. For example, in Chapter 19, Celebrations, the answers for which animals are associated with certain personality traits in the Chinese calendar, are provided on the next page.

- Buying magazines related to the topic you are using can be a great way to add to vocabulary, reading and interaction opportunities.

- Use the internet to search for words related to topics of interest
(be mindful about copyrights when using such material).

CHAPTER 1

THEME: SPRING

CONTENTS				
ACTIVITY & PAGE NUMBER	**ACTIVITY**	**CLIENT GROUP**	**LEVEL**	**COMMENTS & SUGGESTIONS**
1 Pages 2–3	Poem	Speech, voice, fluency, group, language	L2–L3	Page 2 provides suggestions on how to use the poem.
2 Page 4	Naming or discussion activity	All	L1–L3	L1 clients might need written or pictorial prompts.
3 Page 5	Idioms and old wives' tales	All	L2–L3	Good activity to promote discussion.
4(a) Page 6	Crossword – anagrams	Language	L1	
4(b) Page 7	Crossword – clues	Language	L1	
4(c) Page 8	Crossword – answers	Language	L1	
5 Page 9	Spring colours	All	L1–L2	Provide options for clients at L1 to match the colour. To make it harder, you could include options that do not match with any colours given.
6 Page 10	Rhyming words	All	L2–L3	

DOI: 10.4324/9781003177852-1

Activity 1: Poem by William Wordsworth (3 verses)*

I Wandered Lonely as a Cloud

I wander'd lonely as a cloud,
That floats on high o'er vales and hills,
When all at once I saw a crowd,
A host, of golden Daffodils,
Beside the Lake, beneath the trees
Fluttering and dancing in the breeze.

The waves beside them danced, but they
Out-did the sparkling waves in glee:–
A Poet could not but be gay
In such a jocund company!
I gazed – and gazed – but little thought
What wealth the show to me had brought.

For oft, when on my couch I lie
In vacant or in pensive mood,
They flash upon that inward eye
Which is the bliss of solitude;
And then my heart with pleasure fills
And dances with the Daffodils.

Activity 1: Poem

Instructions: This poem can be used in a number of ways:

1) Read it aloud to practise your speech, intonation, voice or fluency.
2) If you are reading aloud, make sure you start with enough air in your lungs to carry your voice.

   Do not strain your voice; take a new breath frequently.
3) Can you find another poem about spring?
4) What do you think about when you read this poem? (spring flowers, past holidays, sunshine, or anything else?)
5) Home practice: find five facts about William Wordsworth or another poet of your choice.
6) Where do you think the poem is set?

*7) This poem actually has four verses. It has been shortened to three for the purpose of this book. Look up the full poem and practise all four verses.

Therapy Targets

Activity 2: Naming or discussion activity

Instructions: Speak or write down your answers for the questions below.

TIP: Use the answers to generate a discussion.

1) Name the spring months:

2) Name five spring flowers:

3) Which festivals or celebrations take place in spring?

4) Describe spring weather:

5) What do you like most about spring?

Therapy Targets

Activity 3: Idioms and old wives' tales

Instructions: Read aloud and discuss these idioms and old wives' tales.

- ❑ Rough winds do shake the darling buds of May.
- ❑ Sweet April showers, do spring May flowers.
- ❑ You are as welcome as the flowers in May.
- ❑ A spring in your step!
- ❑ He's no spring chicken.
- ❑ Don't put all your eggs in one basket.
- ❑ Do not buy a broom, wash a blanket or get married in May.
- ❑ A kind word is like a spring day (Russian proverb).
- ❑ A year is determined by its spring (Portuguese proverb).
- ❑ No matter how long the winter, spring is sure to follow.

Therapy Targets

Activity 4(a): Crossword (anagrams)

Instructions: Unscramble the words to find the answer.

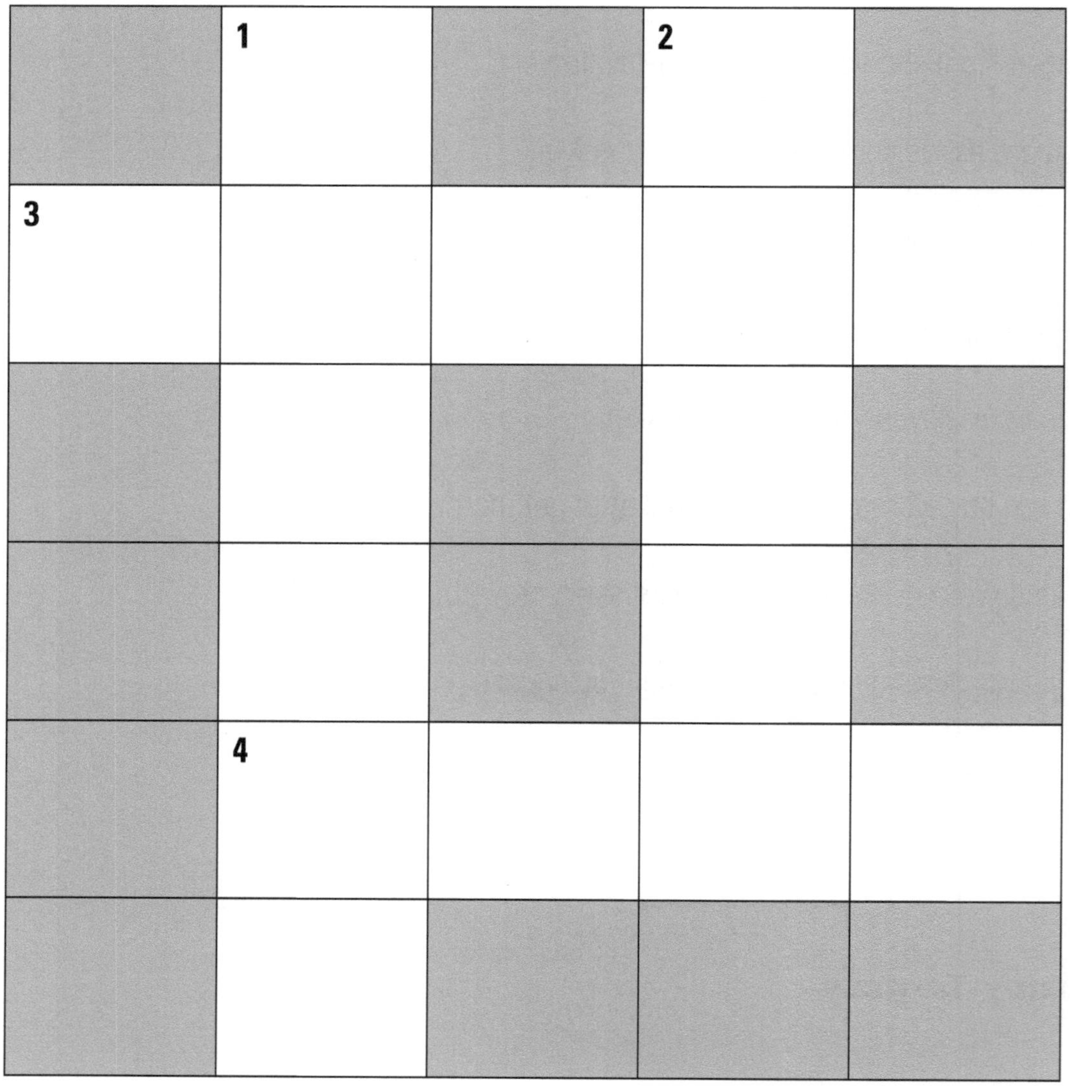

1) P S R N I G

2) B S I D R

3) L A R P I

4) S N E T

Therapy Targets

Activity 4(b): Crossword (clues)

Instructions: Use the clues below to complete the crossword.

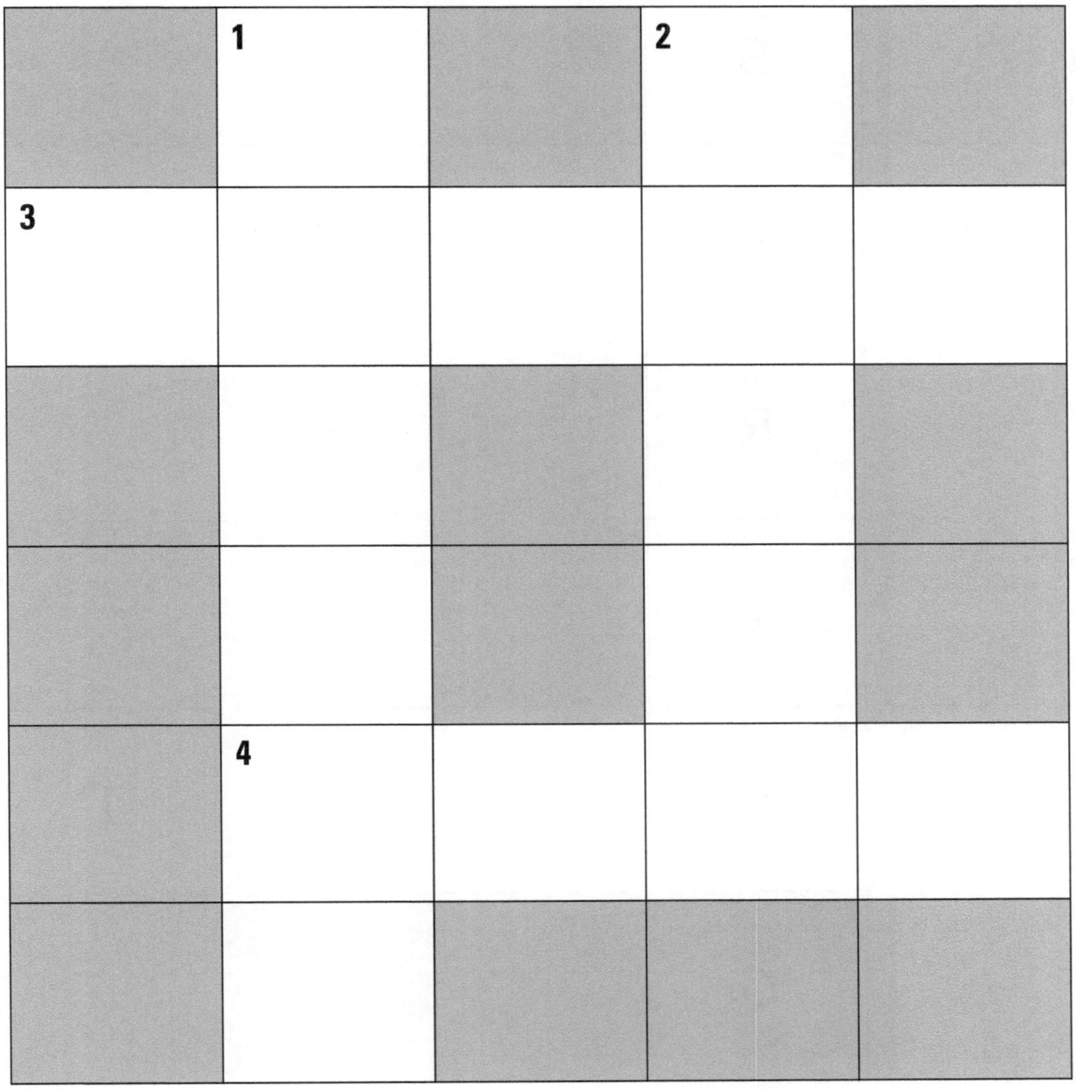

1) First season of the year
2) They build nests
3) Second month of spring
4) Built by birds – in trees and bird boxes

Therapy Targets

Activity 4(c): Crossword (completed)

	1 S		2 B	
3 A	P	R	I	L
	R		R	
	I		D	
	4 N	E	S	T
	G			

Activity 5: Spring colours

Instructions: Take it in turns to roll a dice. Select the colour that matches the number you have rolled. Name something you would see in spring associated with that colour.

Keep going until you cannot think of any more spring-related words.

TIP: This activity could be repeated for each of the seasons.

	Colour
1	Yellow
2	Pink
3	Blue
4	Purple
5	Green
6	White

Therapy Targets

Activity 6: Rhyming words

Instructions: Write or say a word that rhymes with the word in each box. Use the box opposite to write your answer in.

Spring	⇨	
Bird	⇨	
Lamb	⇨	
May	⇨	
Pink	⇨	
Sow	⇨	

Therapy Targets

Activity: Words of increasing length

Instructions: Read across each row. Say the words. Use the words in the third column to make a longer sentence.

The blank boxes at the bottom can be used for your own word sequences.

One syllable	Two syllables	Multisyllabic	Now say a complete sentence using the multisyllabic word or phrase
Nest	Nesting	Nesting birds	
Warm	Warmer	Warmer weather	
Sun	Sunshine	Sunshine and showers	
Flow	Flowers	Spring flowers	
Sow	Sowing	Sowing seeds	
Spring	Springtime	Springtime blossom	

Therapy Targets

CHAPTER 2

THEME: SUMMER

CONTENTS				
ACTIVITY & PAGE NUMBER	**ACTIVITY**	**CLIENT GROUP**	**LEVEL**	**COMMENTS & SUGGESTIONS**
1 Page 14	Ideas-web	All. Especially good for groups and for generating conversation	L2	A selection of pictures with answers could be given to L1 clients, to match to the questions.
2 Page 15	Making sentences	All	L1–L2	
3 Page 16	A summer garden naming task	All	L2–L3	
4 Page 17	Odd-one-out	Speech and language	L2	L3 if client also explains the differences.
5 Page 18	Word to picture matching	Language, especially word recall	L1	
6 Page 19	Anagrams	Language, especially word recall and spelling	L2	
7 Page 20	Holiday phrases	Speech, voice and fluency	L2–L3	
8 Page 21	Talking or writing about a holiday	All	L2–L3	L2 clients might benefit from having written words and pictures provided to convey their ideas.

DOI: 10.4324/9781003177852-2

Activity 1: Ideas-web

Instructions: Answer the questions in the ovals.

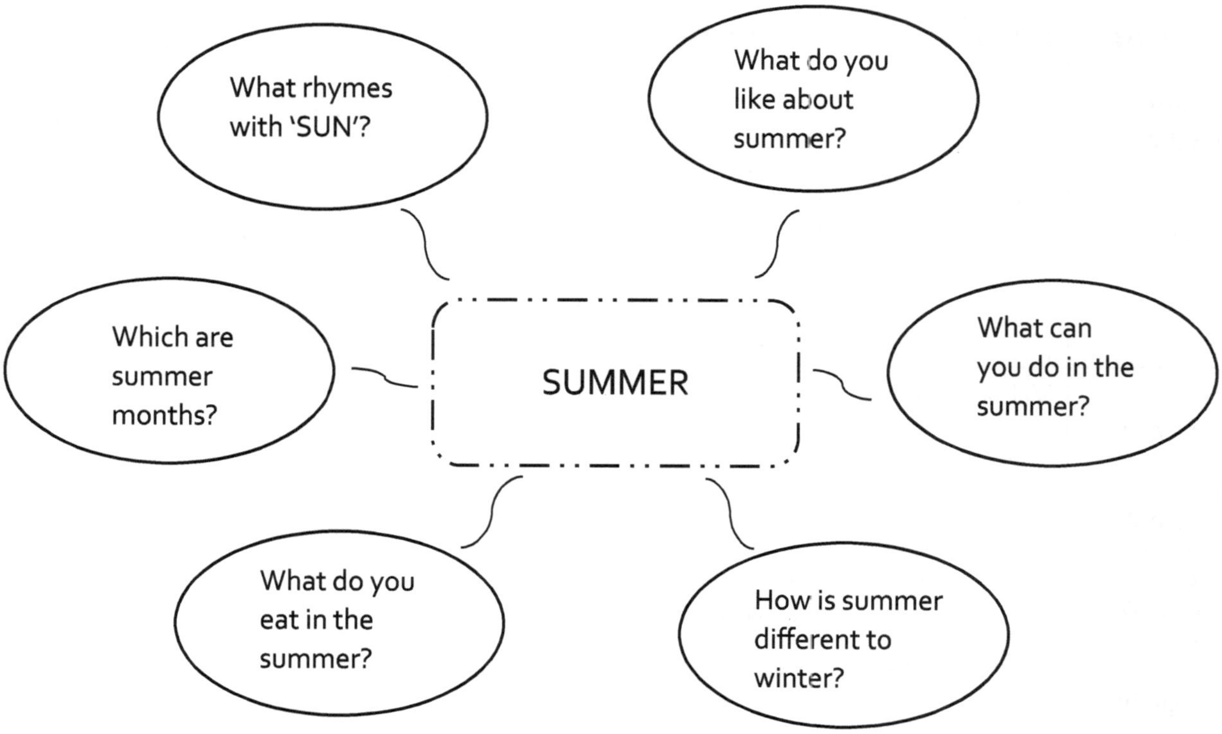

Therapy Targets

Activity 2: Making sentences

Instructions: For each category, roll a dice. Select the word/phrase matching the number on the dice. When you have three words/phrases, arrange them into a sentence.

Category A

1 the man	**4** the girl
2 the dog	**5** the doctor
3 the birds	**6** the ladies

Category B

1 cut	**4** saw
2 dug up	**5** smelt
3 tasted	**6** ate

Category C

1 the flowers	**4** the tree
2 the vegetables	**5** the raspberries
3 the honey	**6** the salad

Do your sentences make sense?

Can you write three more sentences?

Therapy Targets

Activity 3: A summer garden naming task

Instructions: Speak, or write down your answers

Name three summer flowers:

Name three summer birds:

Which flowers do you particularly like?

Which flowers do butterflies like?

Name summer annuals (plants that only flower and live for one season):

Name summer perennials (plants that flower every year):

Therapy Targets

Activity 4: Odd-one-out

Instructions: In each line, which word does not belong to the others? Underline it or say it out loud.

BEES	ANTS	WASPS	BUTTERFLIES
DAISY	ROSE	GERANIUM	SNOWDROP
HOT	COLD	HUMID	SUNNY
SOFA	BENCH	SUNLOUNGER	DECKCHAIR
ROSÉ	PIMM'S	HOT CHOCOLATE	GIN
SCARF	SUNHAT	SHORTS	T-SHIRT
SALAD	BBQ	PICNIC	CASSEROLE

Therapy Targets

Activity 5: Word to picture matching

Instructions: Find the name of each picture in the boxes on the right.

Write your answers next to the picture.

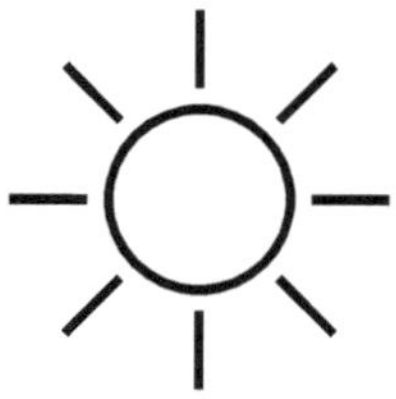

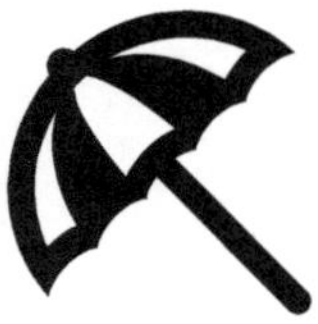

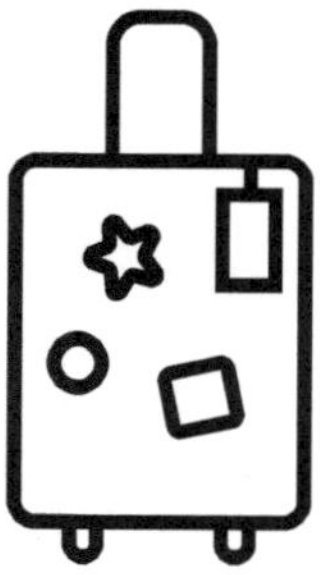

SUNGLASSES
HOLIDAY
FLOWER
SUN-SHADE
SUITCASE
SUN

Therapy Targets

Activity 6: Anagrams

Instructions: Using the letters provided, write the correct word next to each picture.

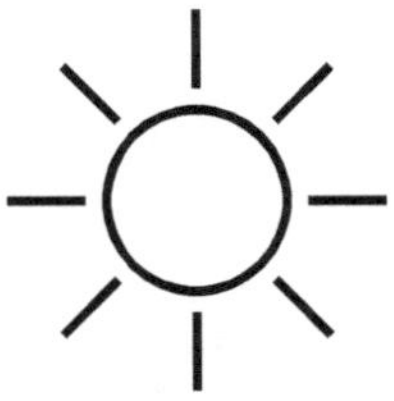

------------------------ N S U

--------------------------- D Y A O I L H

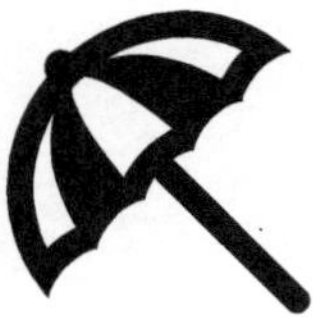

-------------------------------- N U S – D E S A H

------------------------------- R F O L W E

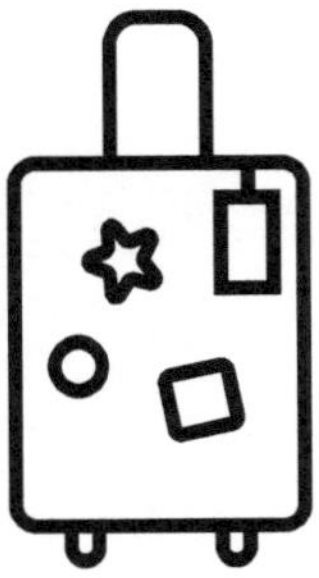

---------------------------------- E C A S U I S T

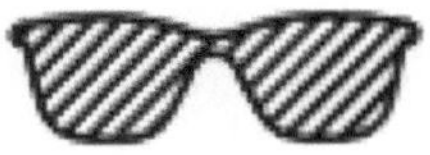

---------------------------------- S L G A S E S S N U

Therapy Targets

Activity 7: Holiday phrases

Instructions: Practise saying these phrases.

What are we doing today?

Time for an ice-cream.

Let's go to the beach.

I'd like to go to the museum.

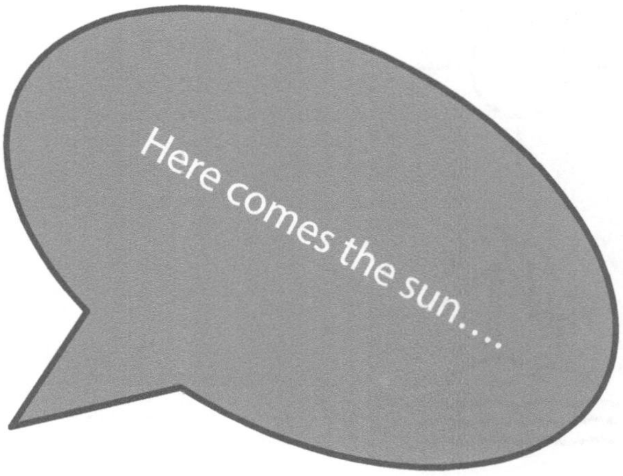

Where's the sun cream?

Where's your sunhat?

Don't forget your sunglasses?

Have you seen my sunglasses?

I've got the map.

Time for a beer.

What an amazing view!

Therapy Targets

Activity 8: Talking or writing about a holiday

Instructions: Think about one of your holidays. Now answer the questions below about that holiday.

When did you go?

What time of year was it?

Where did you go and why?

What type of accommodation did you stay in?

Could you write a short review about it? Would you recommend it, what was the best or worst part, what would you change?

Is there anything else you want to say about it?

Therapy Targets

Activity: Words of increasing length

Instructions: Read across each row. Say the words. Use the words in the third column to make a longer sentence.

The blank boxes at the bottom can be used for your own word sequences.

One syllable	Two syllables	Multisyllabic	Now say a complete sentence using the multisyllabic word or phrase
Buzz	Buzzing	Buzzing bees	
Sun	Sunhat	Sunhat and sunglasses	
Sand	Sandy	Sandy beach	
Sea	Seaside	Seaside air	
Ice	Ice-cream	Vanilla ice-cream	
Hot	Hotter	It's getting hotter	

Therapy Targets

CHAPTER 3

THEME: AUTUMN

CONTENTS				
ACTIVITY & PAGE NUMBER	**ACTIVITY**	**CLIENT GROUP**	**LEVEL**	**COMMENTS & SUGGESTIONS**
1 Page 24	ACROSTICS	All	L2 and L3	Great homework activity, especially in groups, so participants can share their answers.
2 Pages 25–28	Autumn word search 1	Language	L1 and L2	Clues provided at different levels: 2(a) words (page 26), 2(b) anagram & picture (page 27), 2(c) picture only (page 28).
3 and 3(a) Pages 29–30	Autumn word search 2 and ways of using	Language	L1 and L2	Larger grid to increase challenge level.
3(b) Page 31	Autumn word search 2 – word-finding	Language	L1 and L2	Clues for words only. Clients at L2 might need more help to complete. Good for word-finding.
4 Page 32	Poetry – easy poem	All clients	L1 and L3	
5 Page 33	Poetry – longer poem	All clients	L1 and L3	
6 Page 34	Ideas-web (naming association task)	All clients	L2 and L3	Good to promote word recall and naming categories. Can be used in a group to enable controlled turn-taking.
7 Page 35	Sorting words into categories	Language	L2 and L3	With help, some L1 clients might be able to complete this task.

DOI: 10.4324/9781003177852-3

Activity 1: ACROSTICS

Instructions: Use each letter in the word to find a new, related word or phrase. Each new word or phrase begins with each letter of the word provided.

Example: **NUTS**

N – **n**aughty squirrels

U – **u**nearthing bulbs

T – **t**o

S – **s**teal

What words or phrases can you find beginning with each of the letters in '**BERRIES**'.

B

E

R

R

I

E

S

Other words to try:

AUTUMN **LEAF** **RED** **GOLD**

Therapy Targets

Activity 2: Autumn word search 1

Instructions: See Activities 2(a)–2(c) on how to use this letter grid.

A	C	O	R	N	W	E	J
F	L	E	A	F	G	P	U
B	H	A	T	N	R	K	M
T	R	L	A	M	E	H	P
R	I	R	P	H	D	C	E
E	O	K	W	E	A	E	R
E	N	I	K	P	M	U	P
N	B	O	O	T	S	E	S
S	Q	U	I	R	R	E	L

Therapy Targets

Activity 2(a): Clues for autumn word search 1 – words

Instructions: Find these words in the letter grid on page 25.

LEAF

HAT

ACORN

BOOTS

JUMPER

TREE

PUMPKIN

SQUIRREL

Can you find two autumn colours in the word search?

1)

2)

Therapy Targets

Activity 2(b): More clues for autumn word search 1 – anagrams

Instructions: Find these words in the letter grid on page 25.

FAEL 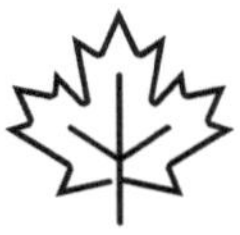

TAH 

ROACN 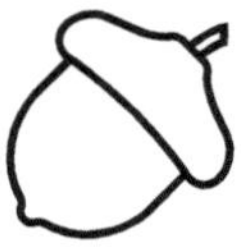

TOBOS 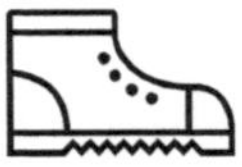

RUMEPJ 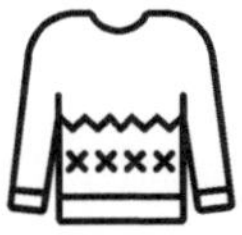

RETE 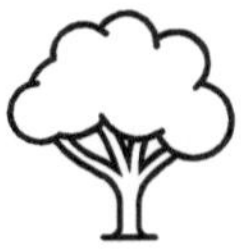

KPMUNIP 

ELSUQIRR 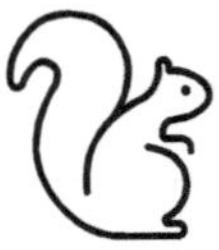

Therapy Targets

Activity 2(c): Clues for autumn word search 1 – pictures

Instructions: Name these pictures. Then find the words on the letter grid on page 25.

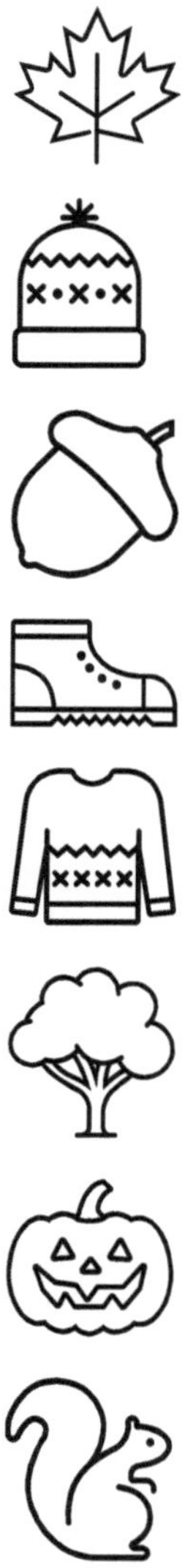

Therapy Targets

Activity 3: Autumn word search 2

Instructions: See Activities 3(a) and 3(b) on how to use this letter grid.

A	C	O	R	B	F	W	E	K	A	E	R	E	E	S	T
N	U	A	O	R	A	N	G	E	H	A	I	C	O	A	T
I	T	T	O	O	E	W	E	A	S	K	C	L	L	E	R
K	K	E	U	P	E	D	D	T	N	A	O	E	O	U	E
P	E	G	L	E	A	F	O	V	B	L	P	R	A	K	E
M	B	R	E	I	U	O	P	S	D	F	P	W	Q	B	C
U	F	D	D	S	B	C	V	W	E	R	E	J	G	D	A
P	N	V	C	X	Z	J	U	M	P	E	R	E	H	A	F
L	G	A	E	A	I	P	I	S	C	S	D	E	A	R	B
B	R	H	T	V	H	D	K	Q	S	S	E	R	T	B	C
F	O	A	E	I	U	O	F	U	B	C	Z	X	M	P	W
E	W	O	S	W	E	L	L	I	E	S	A	C	O	R	N
S	F	D	T	J	N	L	H	R	Y	B	N	S	E	W	R
A	E	F	A	S	M	D	G	R	Y	R	D	V	R	J	E
A	E	I	R	P	K	Y	D	E	H	E	A	B	I	A	E
J	L	N	W	O	R	B	F	L	R	E	T	N	I	I	A

Activity 3(a): Autumn word search 2 – ways of using

Instructions: Look at the letter grid on page 29. See below for ideas on how to use the word search.

Note to therapist: Tick the activity you want your client to do.

- ❑ Use the clues from Activity 2(a).
- ❑ Use the clues from Activity 2(b).
- ❑ Use the clues from Activity 2(c).
- ❑ Answer the questions in Activity 3(b). Now find those words in the word search.
- ❑ Without using any clues, how many autumn words you can find?
- ❑ What other words can you find in the letter grid (that may or may not be related to autumn)?

Therapy Targets

Activity 3(b): Autumn word search 2 – word-finding

Instructions: Read the description in the box below to find the words.

Changes from green to red and falls from the trees	
Wraps around your neck to keep you warm	
The fruit of an oak tree	
Lots of them make a forest	
A warm item of clothing to keep your upper body warm	
Waterproof boots that are made of rubber	
A garden tool for moving fallen leaves into a pile	
The colour of autumnal leaves	

Write or say a sentence from the words you have found.

Can you turn them into a story?

Therapy Targets

Activity 4: Poetry – easy poem

Instructions: Read this poem aloud.

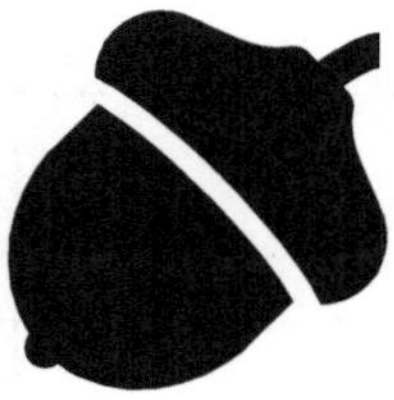

Oak Tree

Ancient oak
Dying leaves
Falling like golden snow

By T B Jackson

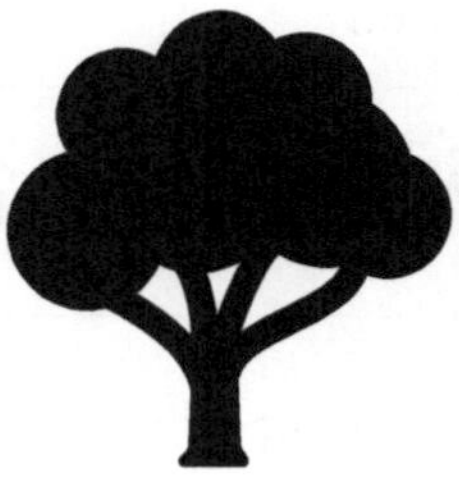

Discussion:

Do you like poetry?

Do you like this poem?

Who is your favourite poet?

Can you write your own poem about autumn?

Therapy Targets

Activity 5: Poetry – longer poem

Instructions: Read this poem aloud.

See page xii in 'How to use this guide' for more therapy ideas.

Digging

To-day I think
Only with scents, – scents dead leaves yield,
And bracken, and wild carrot's seed,
And the square mustard field;

Odours that rise
When the spade wounds the root of tree,
Rose, currant, raspberry, or goutweed,
Rhubarb or celery;

The smoke's smell, too,
Flowing from where bonfire burns
The dead, the waste, the dangerous,
And all to sweetness turns.

It is enough
To smell, to crumble the dark earth,
While the robin sings over again
Sad songs of Autumn mirth.

Philip Edward Thomas (3 March 1878 – 9 April 1917)

Therapy Targets

Activity 6: Ideas-web

Instructions: Answer the questions below about the word 'Pumpkin'.

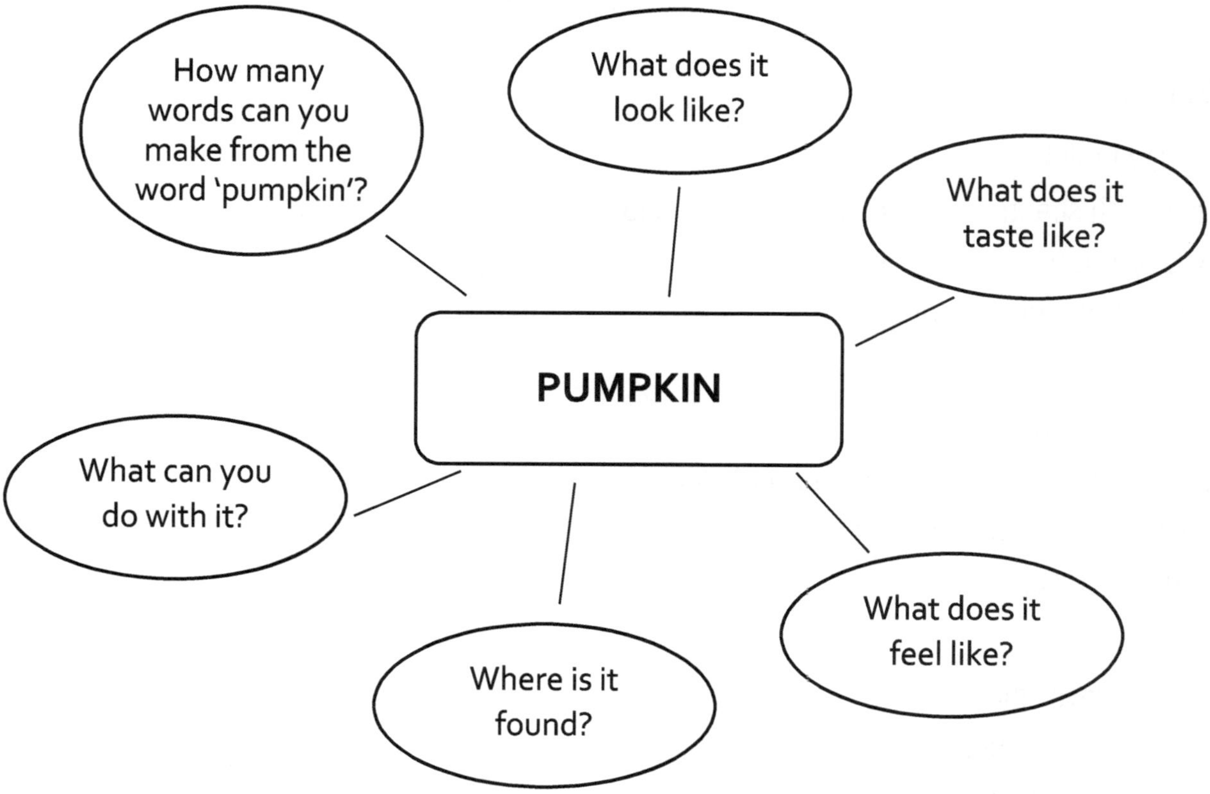

Try this exercise again using these words:

Bonfire

Leaves

Blackberries

Therapy Targets

Activity 7: Sorting words into categories

Instructions: Write the words below next to their correct category. e.g. Fruit – pears.

blackberries	brown	golden	apples	blackberry picking
kicking leaves	bonfire	red	wet leaves	carrot
pear	elderberries	making jam	orange	jacket
potatoes	turnips	long walks	swede	parsnips

Categories

Fruit:

Vegetables:

Colours:

Smells:

Can you think of more words for each category?

Therapy Targets

Activity: Words of increasing length

Instructions: Read across each row. Say the words. Use the words in the third column to make a longer sentence.

The blank boxes at the bottom can be used for your own word sequences.

One syllable	Two syllables	Multisyllabic	Now say a complete sentence using the multisyllabic word or phrase
Fall	Falling	Falling leaves	
Wind	Windy	Windy day	
Fire	Fireworks	Fireworks' display	
Leaf	Leaf fall	Heavy leaf fall	
Fog	Foggy	Foggy morning	
Mist	Misty	Misty day	

Therapy Targets

THEME: WINTER

CONTENTS

DOI: 10.4324/9781003177852-4

Activity 1: Winter plants

Instructions: Name ten winter plants.

TIP: Think about ones that are renowned for their colourful berries, stems, flowers or leaves.

1)

2)

3)

4)

5)

6)

7)

8)

9)

10)

Therapy Targets

Activity 2: Winter birds

Instructions: Name five winter birds.

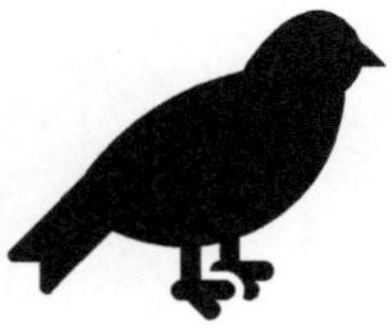

1)

2)

3)

4)

5)

What can you feed birds in the winter?

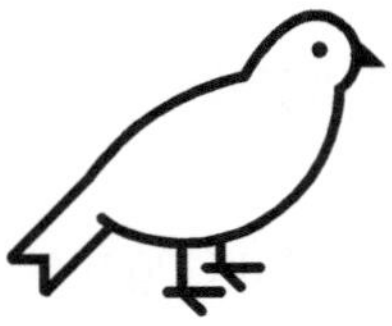

a)

b)

c)

Which is your favourite winter bird?

Therapy Targets

Activity 3(a): Prose 'What is winter?'

Instructions: Read the following prose aloud to practise your speech, voice or fluency strategies.

'What is winter?'

Winter, the coldest season of the year, falls between autumn and spring. The name 'winter' comes from an old Germanic word that means "time of water", referring to the rain and snow of winter in the middle and high latitudes.

In the northern hemisphere, it officially begins with the winter solstice, the year's shortest day. The shortest day is December 21st and winter lasts until the vernal equinox.

The vernal equinox is when day and night are of equal length. The date for this equinox is March 20th. In the southern hemisphere, winter typically falls between June 21st and September 21st. The low temperatures associated with winter bring rain, sleet, snow and ice. Whilst the northern hemisphere is experiencing winter, in the southern hemisphere summer arrives.

Winter is considered to be the season of dormancy and rest. Some plants die after dispersing their seeds, and others merely cease to grow until the relative warmth of spring.

Conversely, some plants come alive in winter, providing stunning colour to the garden. Gardeners' favourites include Mahonia, winter flowering jasmine, snowdrops and hellebores.

Like plants, some animals become dormant in winter and hibernate. Others adapt to the winter months by changing their fur colour. In Britain, hares and ptarmigans (a type of bird) are renowned for this, but animals in other countries also change their fur colour. Some of these are Siberian hamsters, arctic foxes and Peary Caribou (a type of deer). The reason is unknown, but some people believe the colour change creates a camouflage for the animals.

Other theories suggest it is for insulation. There is less melanin in white fur, creating air spaces that provide insulation.

The End

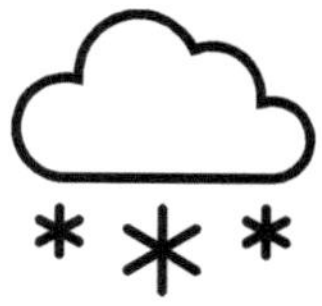

Therapy Targets

Activity 3(b): Questions about the winter prose

Instructions: Ask the client(s) questions about the prose. Here are some example questions.

1) When does winter begin in the northern hemisphere?
2) In which hemisphere is winter from June to September?
3) When does winter end in the northern hemisphere?
4) What do some creatures do in the winter?
5) Name two animals whose fur turns white in the winter.

Discussion:

Do you like winter?

What do you like to do in the winter?

What is your favourite season?

Therapy Targets

Activity 4: Poem – 'I Made a Little Snowman'

Instructions: See page xii in the 'How to use this resource' section for ideas about using this poem.

I Made a Little Snowman

I made a little snowman,
Short and fat and round.
I gave him pebbles for a mouth,
But still he made no sound.

I made a little snowman,
Short and fat and round.
I gave him shoes so he could walk,
But he never left the ground.

I made a little snowman,
Short and fat and round.
I put a hat upon his head,
He looked like he'd been crowned.

I made a little snowman,
Short and fat and round.
I used a carrot for his nose,
But he looked at me and frowned.

I made a little snowman,
Short and fat and round.
I made those pebbles into a smile,
Now his smiles abound.

By T B Jackson, 2021

Therapy Targets

Activity 4(a): Extended activity – snowman

Instructions: Name the different parts of the snowman.

TIP: read the poem first to help recall the words.

Therapy Targets

Activity 5: Rhyming words

Instructions: Can you find a rhyming word for each of the words below?

Example: Snow – glow

Ice

Berry

Frost

Fire

Rain

Cloud

Freeze

Glove

Scarf

December

Fog

Can you make up a poem with these words?

Therapy Targets

Activity 6: Verb (actions) anagrams

Instructions: Unscramble the letters to identify the actions?

g e l s g n i d ________ 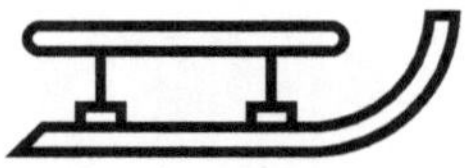

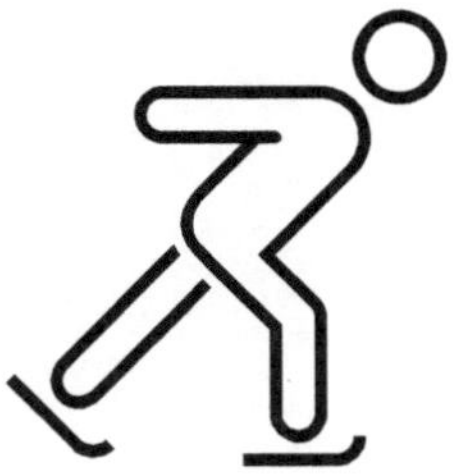

k a s g n i t ________

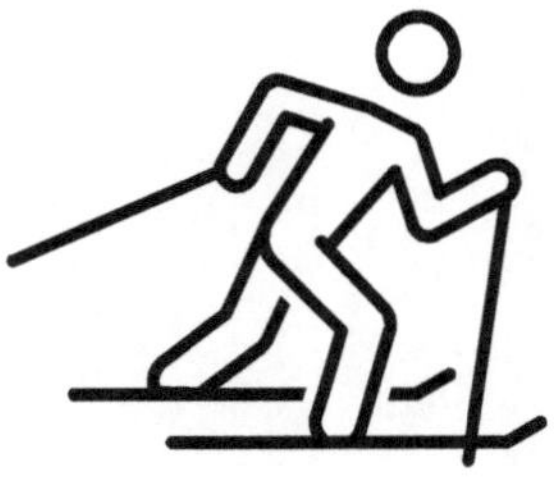

g k s n i i ________

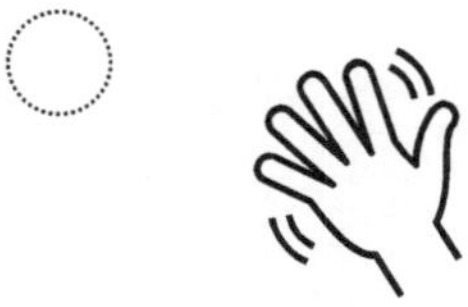

i h r w o t g n (... a snowball) ________

g u l i d n b i (... a snowman) ________

Therapy Targets

Activity 7: Picture to word matching

Instructions: Match the words to the pictures.

Fire

Hot chocolate

Snow

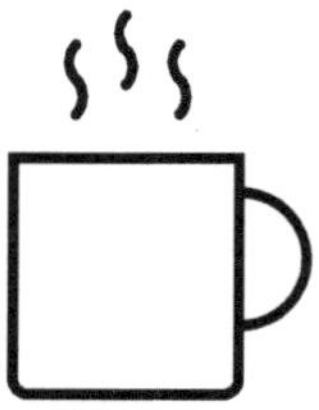

Woolly hat

Snowflake

Freezing

Snowman

Can you put these words into a sentence?

Therapy Targets

Activity 8: Finding smaller words from a longer word

Instructions: How many small words can you find in the long words listed below?

S N O W F L A K E

C H O C O L A T E

F E B R U A R Y

Therapy Targets

Activity 9: Winter sayings and proverbs

Instructions: Read these sayings aloud.

What good is the warmth of summer, without the cold of winter to give it sweetness? *John Steinbeck*

To appreciate the beauty of a snowflake, it is necessary to stand out in the cold. *Aristotle*

Winter is on my head, but eternal spring is in my heart. *Victor Hugo*

Every cloud has a silver lining. *English Proverb*

The fire is winter's fruit. *Arabian Proverb*

They who sing through summer, must dance in the winter. *Italian Proverb*

One kind word can warm three winter months. *Japanese Proverb*

Can you find any more winter sayings?

Therapy Targets

Activity: Words of increasing length

Instructions: Read across each row. Say the words. Use the words in the third column to make a longer sentence.

The blank boxes at the bottom can be used for your own word sequences.

One syllable	Two syllables	Multisyllabic	Now say a complete sentence using the multisyllabic word or phrase
Pine	Pinecones	Pinecones falling	
Snow	Snowflakes	Snowflakes melting	
Cold	Colder	Colder weather	
Frost	Frosty	Frosty morning	
Freeze	Freezing	Freezing cold	
Ice	Icy	Icy wind	

Therapy Targets

CHAPTER 5

THEME: FILMS

CONTENTS				
ACTIVITY & PAGE NUMBER	**ACTIVITY**	**CLIENT GROUP**	**LEVEL**	**COMMENTS & SUGGESTIONS**
1(a) Page 52	Film titles – spoken	All	L1–L3	Good warm up activity for a group or individual session.
1(b) Page 53	Film titles – written	Language	L2–L3	
2 Page 54	Famous film actors	All	L1–L3	Good warm up activity for a group or individual session.
3 Page 55	Favourite films	All	L2–L3	Use where client needs to produce continuous speech; good group activity.
4(a) Page 56	Word association	Language	L2–L3	Good for groups. Clients could work in pairs then compare lists.
4(b) Page 57	Word association – with picture clues	Language	L1–L2	Ask client to match written word to picture.
5(a) Page 58	Word association – action words	Language	L3	With some extra clues, could be a L2 task, e.g. give first letter.
5(b)–(c) Pages 59–60	Word association – action words answers, further suggestions and blank activity sheet	All	L2–L3	Blank sheet provided for flexible presentation of this activity.
6 Page 61	Comparisons	All	L1–L3	For L1 clients, use pictures.
7 Page 62	Verbal reasoning (pros and cons)	All	L1–L3	Provide pictures to support L1 and L2.
8 Page 63	Film genre word search	All	L1–L3	Provide clues according to client level.

DOI: 10.4324/9781003177852-5

Activity 1(a): Film titles – spoken activity

Instructions: Complete these famous film titles. Read the first part of the film for your client to complete.

The Lion ___________	(King)
Singing in the ___________	(Rain)
Return of the ___________	(Jedi)
Forrest ___________	(Gump)
Silence of the ___________	(Lambs)
One Flew over the ___________	(Cuckoo's Nest)
Saving Private ___________	(Ryan)
Schindler's ___________	(List)
Gone with the ___________	(Wind)
Lord of the ___________	(Rings)
Back to the ___________	(Future)
Raiders of the ___________	(Lost Ark)
Quantum of ___________	(Solace)
Casino ___________	(Royale)

Therapy Targets

Activity 1(b): Film titles – written activity

Instructions: Can you complete the film title? Write it down.

The Lion ___________

Singing in the ___________

Return of the ___________

Forrest ___________

Silence of the ___________

One Flew over the ___________

Saving Private___________

Schindler's___________

Gone with the ___________

Lord of the ___________

Back to the ___________

Raiders of the ___________

Quantum of ___________

Casino ___________

Therapy Targets

Activity 2: Famous film actors

Instructions: In which films did these actors appear? This can be completed as a spoken or written exercise.

Judy Dench

Arnold Schwarzenegger

Meryl Streep

Jonny Depp

Clint Eastwood

Harrison Ford

Helen Mirren

Liam Neeson

Samuel L Jackson

Maggie Smith

Daniel Craig

Angelina Jolie

Katherine Zeta-Jones

Extra activity:

Who is your favourite actor? Which is your favourite film they starred in?

Therapy Targets

Activity 3: Favourite films

Instructions: Write or talk about your favourite film.

TIP: See the list below for hints of what to think about:

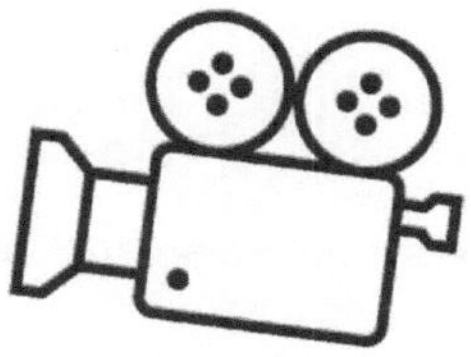

- ❑ The title
- ❑ The characters
- ❑ The plot
- ❑ What is the setting?
- ❑ Why is it your favourite?

Therapy Targets

Activity 4(a): Word association – no clues

Instructions: Write down or talk about other words you recall when you think about the word 'cinema'.

CINEMA

Therapy Targets

Activity 4(b): Word association – picture clues

Instructions: Write down or talk about other words you recall when you think about the word 'cinema'.

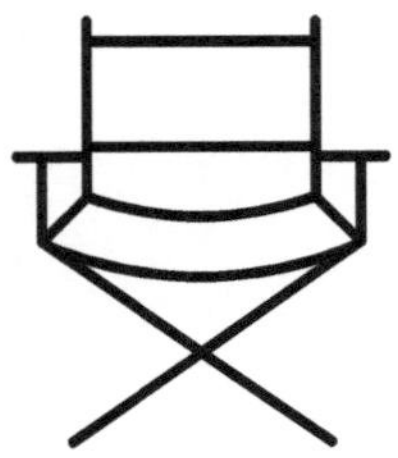
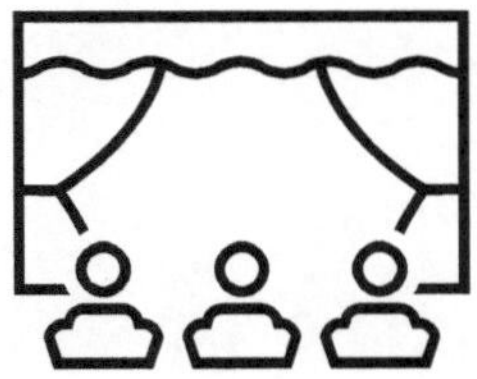
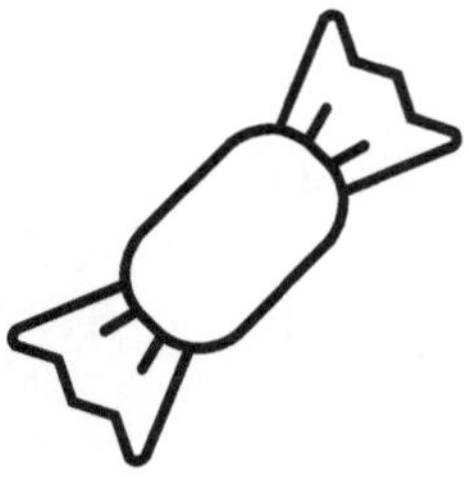

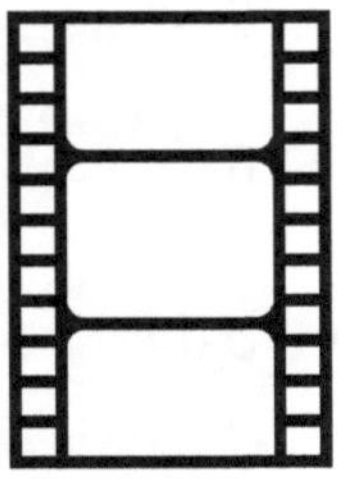

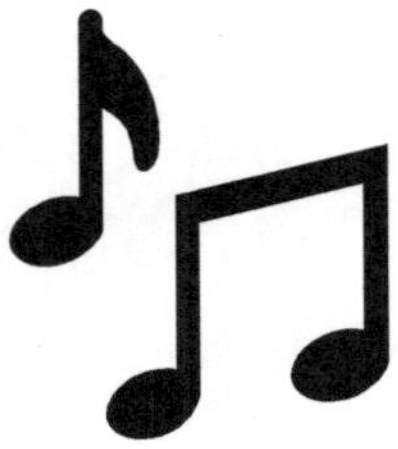
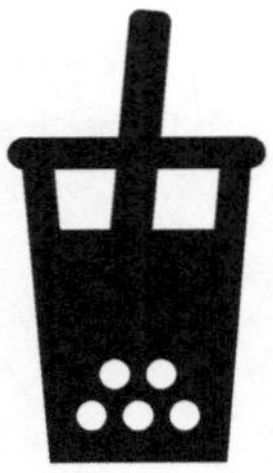
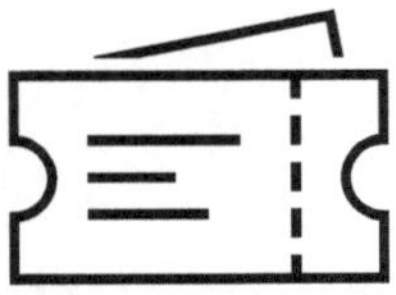

Therapy Targets

Activity 5(a): Word association – action words

Instructions: Unscramble these anagrams to find the action words associated with the word 'cinema'.

c t i a g n

d u r i p o c g n

t w a c h n g i

r t e n d i c i g n

g f i i l m n

d t i g e i n

n a i t i u o d

r p o r e m n i g f

g n r e i v w i e

Therapy Targets

Activity 5(b): Word association – action words

Answers to the anagrams:

c t i a g n	(acting)
d u r i p o c g n	(producing)
t w a c h n g i	(watching)
r t e n d i c i g n	(directing)
g f i i l m n	(filming)
d t i g e i n	(editing)
n a i t i u o d	(audition)
r p o r e m n i g f	(performing)
g n r e i v w i e	(reviewing)

Alternative suggestions:

Use the **blank page overleaf** to write out your own worksheet.

- ❑ Provide the client with the first letter of the word to help unscramble the anagram
- ❑ Provide the word with a missing letter (or two)
- ❑ Write out the words to be spoken for multisyllabic speech practice
- ❑ Ask the client to produce a sentence using one or more of the action words
- ❑ Ask the client to write adverbs for each of the verbs

Therapy Targets

Activity 5(c): Word association – action words

Instructions:

Therapy Targets

Activity 6: Comparisons

Instructions: Describe (by speaking or writing) the similarities and differences between the terms below.

Cinema	Theatre
Film	Play
T.V. series	Film
Action film	Romance
Documentary	Film
Comedy	Thriller
Actor	Performer
Popcorn	Sweets

Therapy Targets

Activity 7: Verbal reasoning (pros and cons)

Instructions: Discuss the pros and cons of watching a film at home versus at the cinema.

Films at home 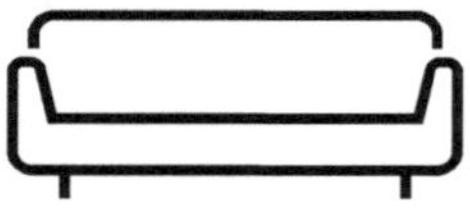	Films at the cinema 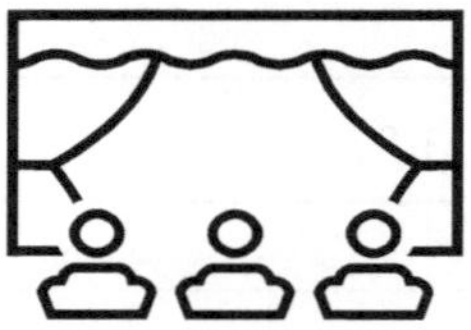
PROS	
CONS	

Therapy Targets

Activity 8: Film genre word search

Instructions: Find the words below in the letter grid.

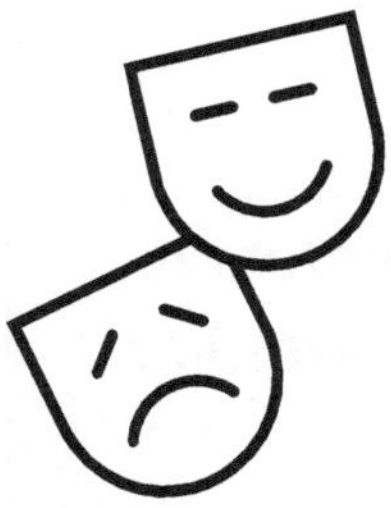

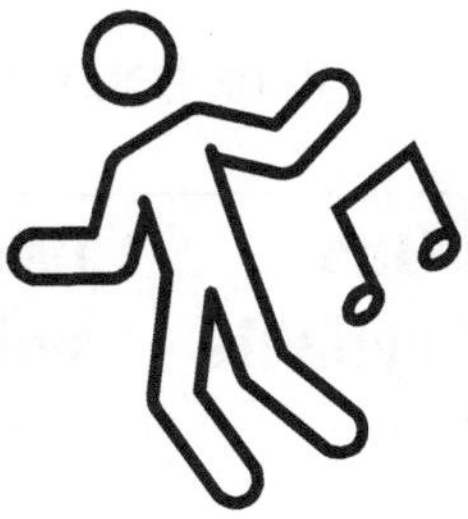

D	D	H	R	O	R	R	O	H
O	C	R	A	N	S	V	R	I
R	O	M	A	N	C	E	Y	S
E	M	D	S	M	L	D	B	T
W	E	O	C	L	A	G	I	O
K	D	I	I	P	J	L	E	R
T	Y	R	F	C	W	G	H	I
I	H	A	I	E	M	I	R	C
T	S	Z	M	R	Q	U	I	A
M	U	S	I	C	A	L	A	L
A	D	V	E	N	T	U	R	E

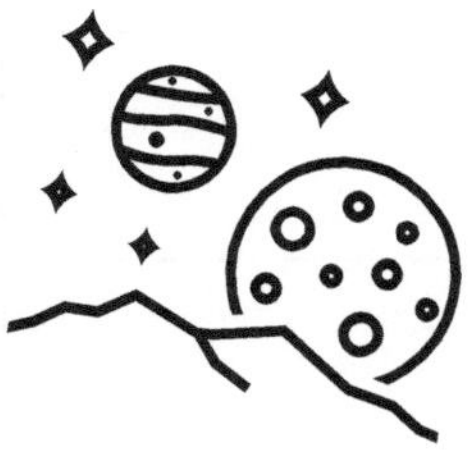

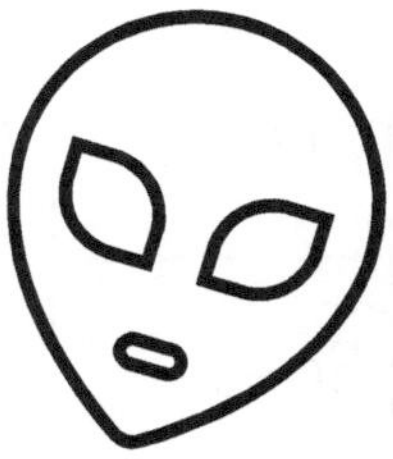

ADVENTURE

HISTORICAL

DRAMA

CRIME

SCI-FI

HORROR

MUSICAL

COMEDY

THRILLER

ROMANCE

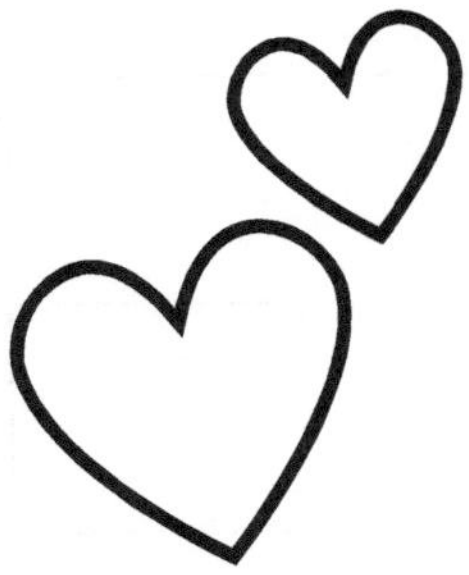

Therapy Targets

Activity: Words of increasing length

Instructions: Read across each row. Say the words. Use the words in the third column to make a longer sentence.

The blank boxes at the bottom can be used for your own word sequences.

One syllable	Two syllables	Multisyllabic	Now say a complete sentence using the multisyllabic word or phrase
Pop	Popcorn	Toffee popcorn	
Act	Action	Action film	
Screen	Screenplay	Screenplay writer	
Prod	Produce	Producer	
Act	Actor	Famous actor	
Trail	Trailer	Watch the trailer	

Therapy Targets

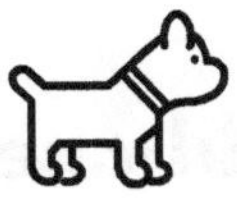
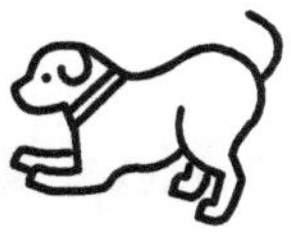

CHAPTER 6

THEME: DOGS

CONTENTS				
ACTIVITY & PAGE NUMBER	**ACTIVITY**	**CLIENT GROUP**	**LEVEL**	**COMMENTS & SUGGESTIONS**
1(a) Page 66	Odd-one-out	Language	L1	Make into a L2–L3 activity – ask the client to explain their answer.
1(b) Page 67	Odd-one-out	Language	L2–L3	
2(a) Page 68	Limerick	Speech, language, fluency, voice	L2–L3	
2(b) Page 69	Limerick	Speech, language, fluency, voice	L2–L3	
3 Page 70	Naming dog body parts	Language, Speech, group	L1–L2	Clients at L1 might need some help.
4 Page 71	Verb (actions) anagrams	Language, Group	L2	
5 Pages 72–73	Dog categorisation	Language, Speech, group	L2	There might be more than one answer. Encourage group discussion to explore possible answers.
6 Page 74	Word retrieval board game	Language, speech, group	L2–L3	With picture cues, could be adapted for L1.
7 Page 75	Tell us about a dog you know	Speech, language, fluency, voice, group	L1–L3	L1 will require some help to select appropriate words, pictures, gestures.

DOI: 10.4324/9781003177852-6

Activity 1(a): Odd-one-out

Instructions: For each row, identify which word doesn't belong with the others.

labrador	spaniel	door	poodle
collar	tree	harness	lead
ball	frisbee	soft toy	sky
house	walk	jump	run
paw	car	tail	ears
bark	dig	knit	sniff
sit	stay	come	write

Therapy Targets

Activity 1(b): Odd-one-out

Instructions: For each row, identify which word doesn't belong with the others.

Labrador	Spaniel	Poodle	Siamese
collar	harness	bone	muzzle
lead	ball	frisbee	soft toy
walk	fly	jump	run
wings	paw	tail	claw
Rottweiler	Doberman	Poodle	Alsatian
Jack Russell	St. Bernard's	Pug	Dachshund

Therapy Targets

Activity 2(a): Limerick

Instructions: Read this limerick aloud.

Coco Loco

There once was a dog called Coco!
Who'd tear round the lounge going loco
She loved chasing her ball
From the bedroom to the hall
That crazy little dog called Coco!

Darren Kinnersley-Hill (2019)

Discussion

What sort of dog do you think Coco is?

Is she young or old?

What was her favourite toy?

What else do you think she enjoys doing?

Therapy Targets

Activity 2(b): Limerick

Instructions: Read this limerick aloud.

Serious!

There once was a dog named Serious,
Who thought he was rather imperious.
He chased sheep in the snow,
Who turned round and said 'No!',
And now he's feeling more spurious.

T B Jackson (2021)

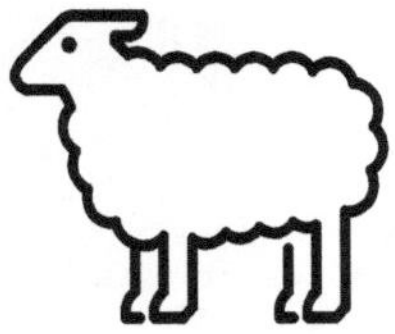

1) Try writing a limerick about a dog you know?

2) What do the words 'serious', 'imperious' and 'spurious' mean?

Therapy Targets

Activity 3: Naming dog body parts

Instructions: Name these dog body parts.

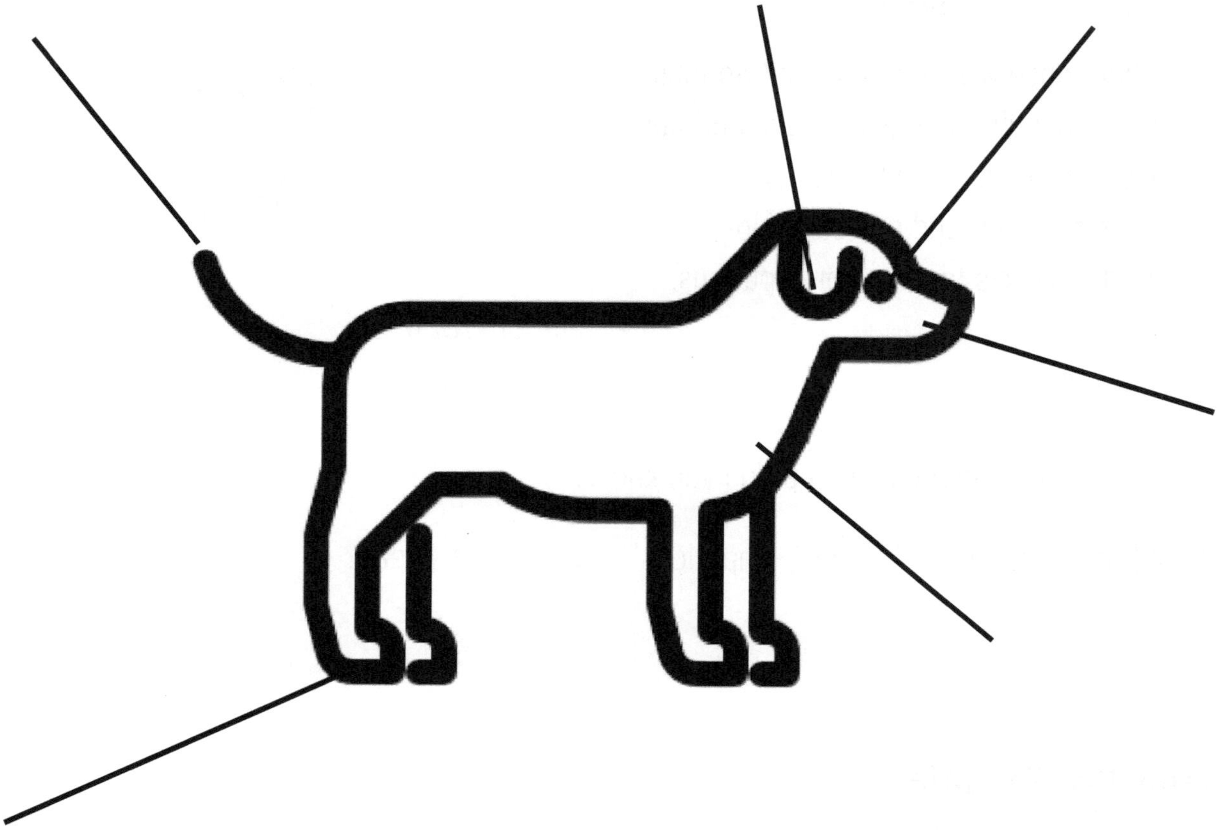

Can you name any other parts?

Therapy Targets

Activity 4: Verb (actions) anagrams

Instructions: Unscramble the anagrams to find words describing actions that dogs do.

T I S

L P Y A

I G D

E C H S A

R N U

F N F I S

K B R A

P E L E S

T A E

H C W E

W S M I

Therapy Targets

Activity 5: Dog categorisation

Instructions: What do these dogs have in common?

BREED	What do they have in common?
Labrador, Golden Retriever, Newfoundland	
Alsatian, Rottweiler, Doberman	
St. Bernard, Pyrenean, Bernese	
Cockerpoo, Labradoodle, Caverpoo	
Cavalier, Springer, Cocker	
Yorkshire, Airedale, Staffordshire	
Boston Terrier, Chesapeake Bay Retriever, American Eskimo Dog	
Collies, Corgis, Kelpies, Heelers	
Miniature Schnauzer, Dachshund, French Bulldog	

Therapy Targets

Suggested answers for Activity 5: Dog categorisation

NB: There might be more than one commonality.

BREED	What do they have in common?
Labrador, Golden Retriever, Newfoundland	Water-loving dogs
Alsatian, Rottweiler, Doberman	Often associated as guard dogs, especially in films
St. Bernard, Pyrenean, Bernese	Mountain dogs
Cockerpoo, Labradoodle, Caverpoo	Poodle crossbreeds
Cavalier, Springer, Cocker	Spaniels
Yorkshire, Airedale, Staffordshire	Terriers Named after counties/areas in England
Boston Terrier, Chesapeake Bay Retriever, American Eskimo Dog	Dogs originating from the USA
Collies, Corgis, Kelpies, Heelers	Dogs bred for their ability to herd sheep and cattle
Miniature Schnauzer, Dachshund, French Bulldog	Small dogs

Therapy Targets

Activity 6: Word retrieval board game

Instructions: Play the board game by following the instructions on the board to recall words. Take a rest on the circles or feel free to add your own activity such as a gesture, speech sound, word or more questions.

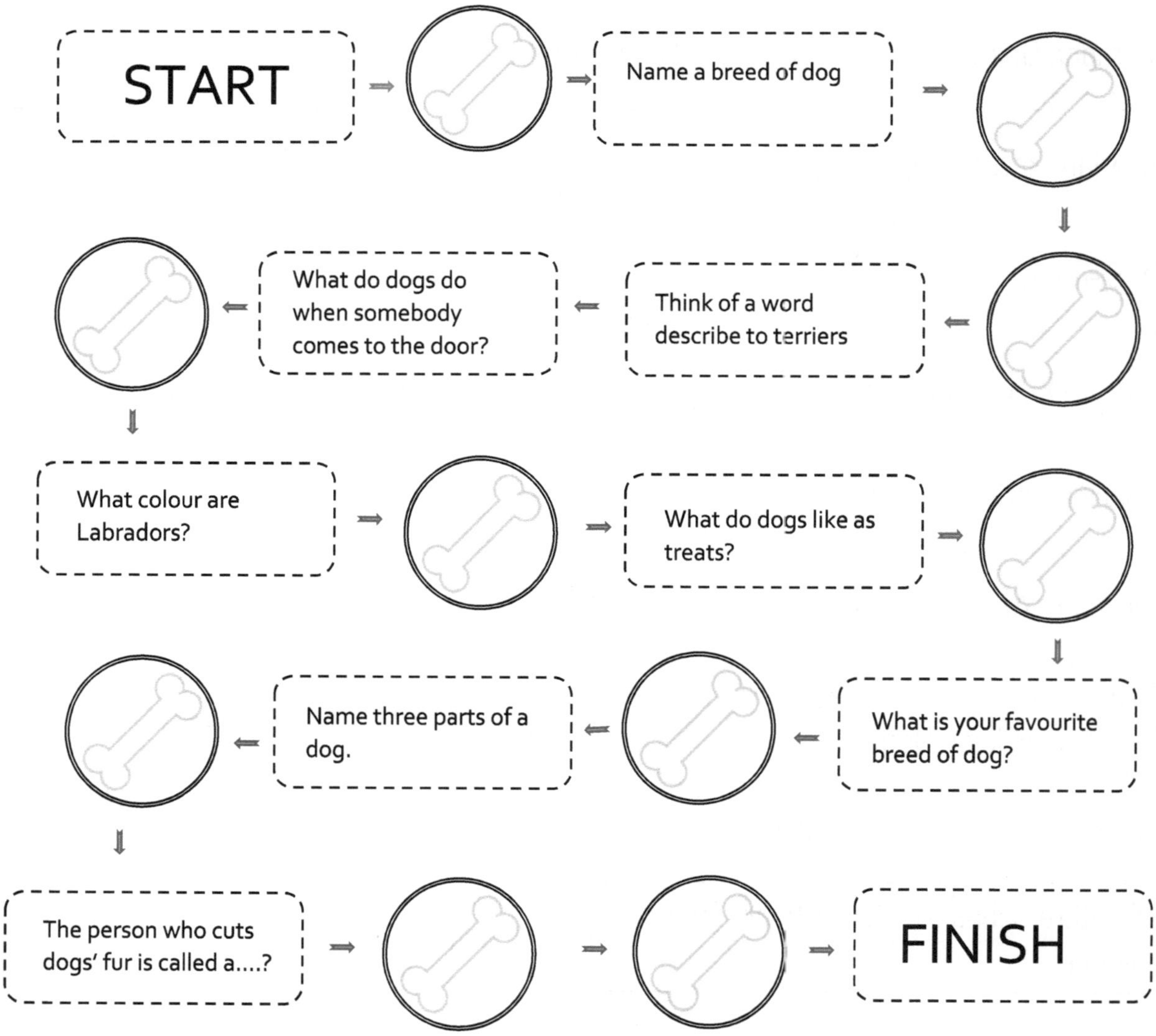

Therapy Targets

Activity 7: Tell us about a dog you know

Instructions: Prepare to tell me/us about a particular dog.

It might be your favourite breed of dog, a dog you own, a dog you have owned, a friend or relative's dog.

TIP: Think about their breed, appearance, personality and favourite treat.

Therapy Targets

Activity: Words of increasing length

Instructions: Read across each row. Say the words. Use the words in the third column to make a longer sentence.

The blank boxes at the bottom can be used for your own word sequences.

One syllable	Two syllables	Multisyllabic	Now say a complete sentence using the multisyllabic word or phrase
Lead	Leading	Leading astray	
Pant	Panting	Panting dog	
Feed	Feeding	Feeding the dog	
Chew	Chewing	Chewing the shoe	
Chase	Chasing	Chasing the cat	
Stroke	Stroking	Stroking the dogs	

Therapy Targets

CHAPTER 7

THEME: CATS

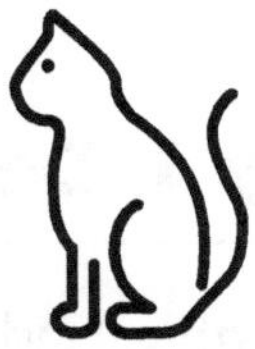

CONTENTS				
ACTIVITY & PAGE NUMBER	**ACTIVITY**	**CLIENT GROUP**	**LEVEL**	**COMMENTS & SUGGESTIONS**
1 Page 78	Describing words	Language, group	L1–L2	
2 Page 79	Writing sentences	Language, speech, fluency	L2–L3	
3 Page 80	Words beginning with 'cat'	Language, speech, Group	L2–L3	
4(a) Page 81	Naming the big cats	Language, speech, Group	L2	
4(b) Page 82	Naming big cats – anagrams	Language	L2–L3	
5 Page 83	Cat sayings	Language, speech, fluency, voice	L2–L3	
6 Page 84	Word to picture matching	Language	L1	Make the task harder by covering up the words or asking the client to put the words into a sentence.
7 Page 85	ACROSTICS	Language, speech, voice	L2–L3	For L1 clients, write words for them, ask them to the word to the letter.

DOI: 10.4324/9781003177852-7

Activity 1: Describing words

Instructions: Underline the words that might describe cats.

licking | fly | clumsy | sleeping

leaping | furry | spikey

graceful | reptile | calm | prowl

territorial | agile

tabby | stalking | square

four-legged | nine lives

Therapy Targets

Activity 2: Writing sentences

Instructions: Use the words from Activity 1 to write some sentences.

1)

2)

3)

4)

5)

6)

Therapy Targets

Activity 3: Words beginning with 'cat'

Instructions: Can you think of words that begin with the syllable 'cat'. They do not have to be cat-related words.

Example:

*Cat*apult

Therapy Targets

Activity 4(a): Naming the big cats

Instructions: How many of the big cats can you name?

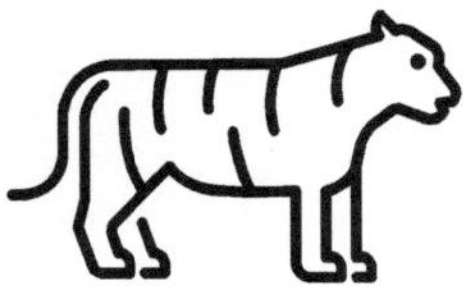

List any big cats you know:

1)

2)

3)

4)

5)

6)

Write down or say three characteristics of the big cats:

i)

ii)

iii)

Therapy Targets

Activity 4(b): Naming the big cats – anagrams

Instructions: Unscramble the letters to spell these big cats. Write your answers in the empty boxes.

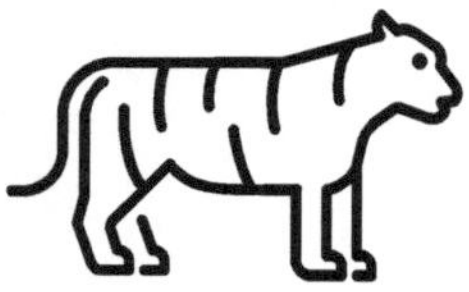

a j u g r a

h h t e e c a

n i l o

p o e l r d a

g t i r e

r c g u a o

Therapy Targets

Activity 5: Cat sayings

Instructions: Practise saying these quotes aloud.

- ❑ While the rest of the species is descended from apes, redheads are descended from cats. *Mark Twain*[1]
- ❑ What greater gift than the love of a cat? *Charles Dickens*[1]
- ❑ The smallest feline is a masterpiece. *Leonardo da Vinci*[1]
- ❑ I believe cats to be spirits come to earth; a cat, I am sure, could walk on a cloud without coming through. *Jules Verne*[1]
- ❑ It is a very inconvenient habit of kittens (Alice once made the remark) that, whatever you say to them, they always purr. *Lewis Carroll*[2]
- ❑ Curiosity killed the cat, satisfaction brought it back. *Old Proverb*

[1] *Cats Quotes (1070 quotes) (goodreads.com)*

[2] *Through the Looking-Glass - Chapter 12 (cleavebooks.co.uk)*

Can you find more quotes about cats?

Therapy Targets

Activity 6: Word to picture matching

Instructions: Write the correct word next to the picture.

NB: There are more words than pictures.

CAT	MOUSE	PAW PRINTS	LICK
TIGER	WOOL / YARN	COMB	KITTEN

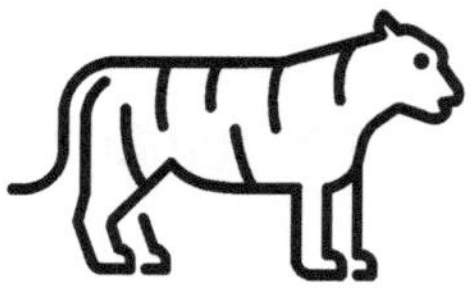
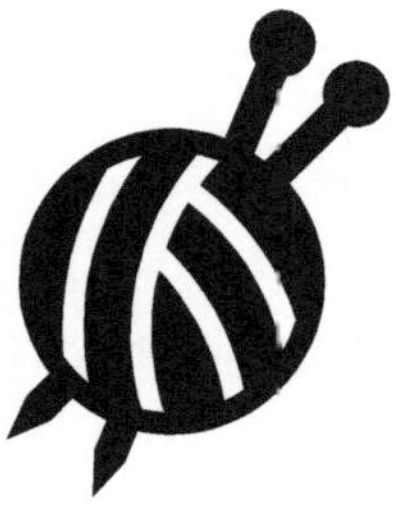
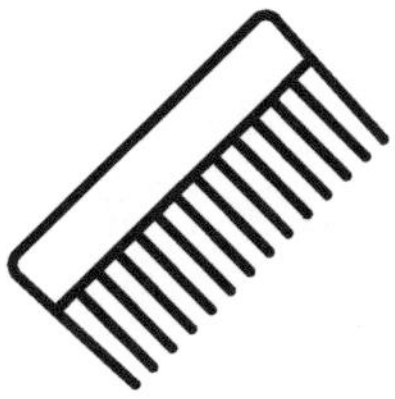
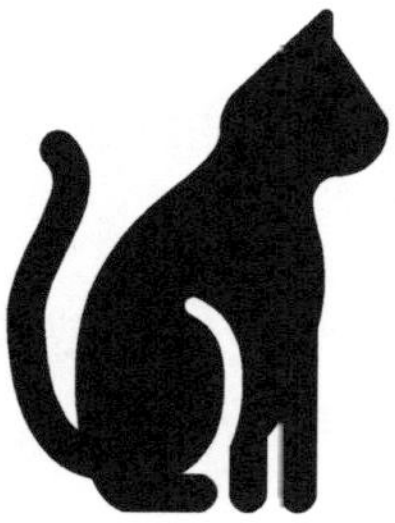
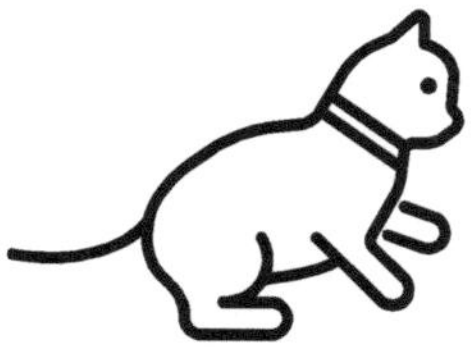
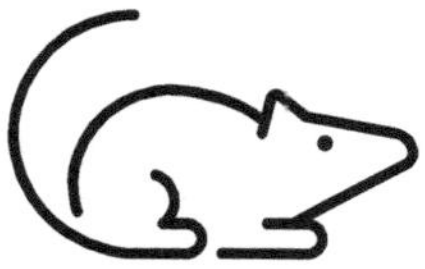

Therapy Targets

Activity 7: ACROSTICS

Instructions: Use each letter in the word to find new, related words or a phrase. Each new word or phrase begins with each letter of the given word.

For example:

C – **c**alm
A – **a**gile
T – **t**ame

Now do your own:

C

A

T

****

K

I

T

T

E

N

****

F

E

L

I

N

E

Therapy Targets

Activity: Words of increasing length

Instructions: Read across each row. Say the words. Use the words in the third column to make a longer sentence.

The blank boxes at the bottom can be used for your own word sequences.

One syllable	Two syllables	Multisyllabic	Now say a complete sentence using the multisyllabic word or phrase
Chase	Chasing	Chasing a mouse	
Lap	Lapping	Lapping up the milk	
Stroke	Stroking	Stroking the cat	
Purr	Purring	Purring loudly	
Knead	Kneading	Kneading the pillow	
Claw	Clawing	Clawing the sofa	

Therapy Targets

CHAPTER 8

THEME: TRAVEL

CONTENTS				
ACTIVITY & PAGE NUMBER	ACTIVITY	CLIENT GROUP	LEVEL	COMMENTS & SUGGESTIONS
1 Page 88	Everyday phrases	Speech, language, voice, fluency	L2–L3	For L1 clients, highlight and practise a keyword, or ask the person to say the last word in the sentence.
2 Page 89	Complete the phrase	All	L1–L3	
3 Page 90	Ideas-web: aeroplane	Speech, language	L2–L3	
4 Page 91	Holiday review	All	L1–L3	L1: Use pictures and sort into 'things I enjoyed' and 'things I didn't enjoy'.
5 Page 92	Guess the city	All	L2–L3	Especially good for groups.
6 Page 93	Finding smaller words from longer words	Language, group	L2–L3	
7 Page 94	Travel words	Language	L1–L2	
8 Page 95	Odd-one-out	Language	L2–L3	
9(a) Page 96	Categories	All	L2–L3	
9(b) Page 97	Categories – words provided	Language	L1	
10 Page 98	What type of holiday?	All	L2–L3	
11 Page 99	The eco-friendly traveller	All	L1–L3	Use pictures to support L1 clients.

DOI: 10.4324/9781003177852-8

Activity 1: Everyday phrases

Instructions: Practise saying these phrases.

What are we doing today?

Time for an ice cream!

Let's go to the beach.

I'd like to go to the museum.

Have you put some sun cream on?

Where's the sun cream?

Where's your sunhat?

Don't forget your sunglasses?

Have you seen my sunglasses?

I've got the map.

Time for a beer!

What an amazing view!

Write 3 of your own phrases:

1)

2)

3)

Therapy Targets

Activity 2: Complete the phrase

Instructions: Write or speak the phrase using your own words.

What are we doing ....?

Time for ....

Let's go to the ....

I fancy going to the ....

Where's the ....?

What a wonderful ....

Don't forget your ....

Therapy Targets

Activity 3: Ideas-web

Instructions: Answer the questions in the ovals below. Your answers should relate to the word 'aeroplane'.

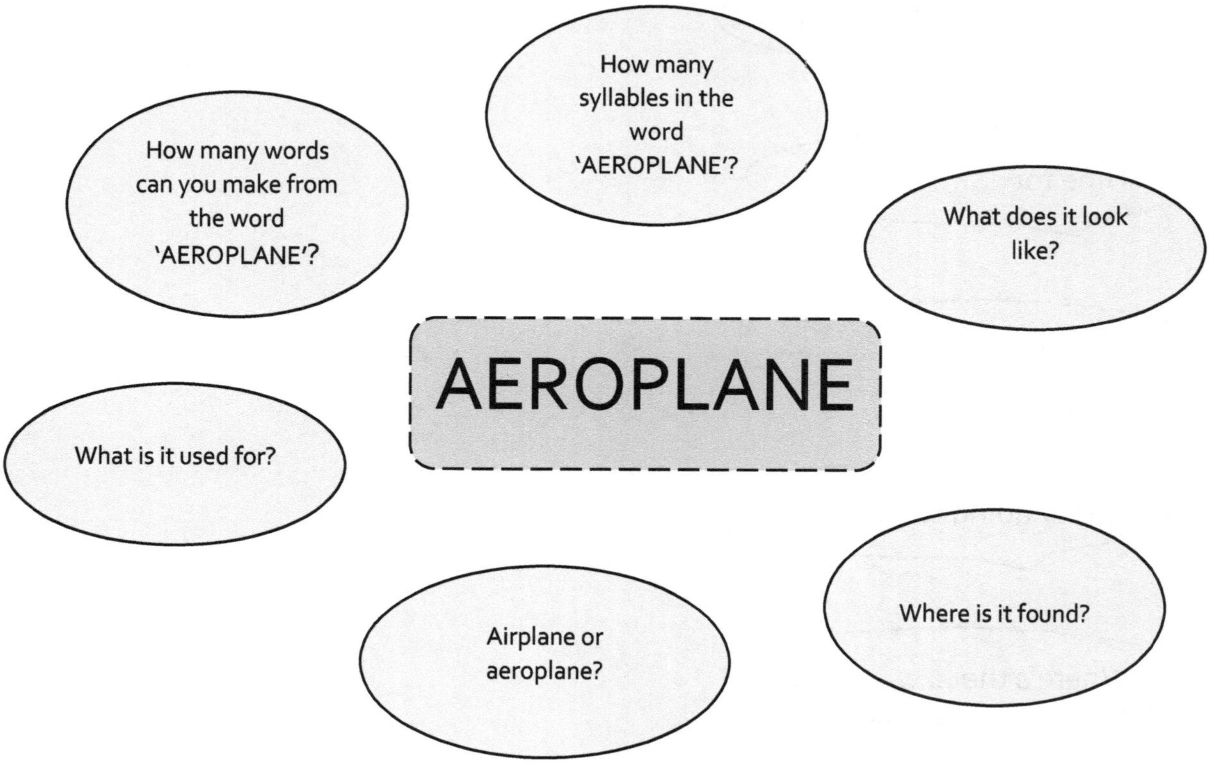

Therapy Targets

Activity 4: Holiday review

Instructions: Think of a holiday you have been on. Use the questions below to help you describe it.

Where did you go?

Why did you go there?

Where did you stay; what sort of accommodation did you stay in?

Would you recommend the accommodation?

Would you recommend the resort?

What was the best or worst part?

What would you change about the holiday?

Therapy Targets

Activity 5: Guess the city (or country)

Instructions: Guess the city or country from the clues.

1) Think of a town, city or country.
2) Describe it so others can guess which town, city or country you are describing.
3) Try not to name it as you describe it!

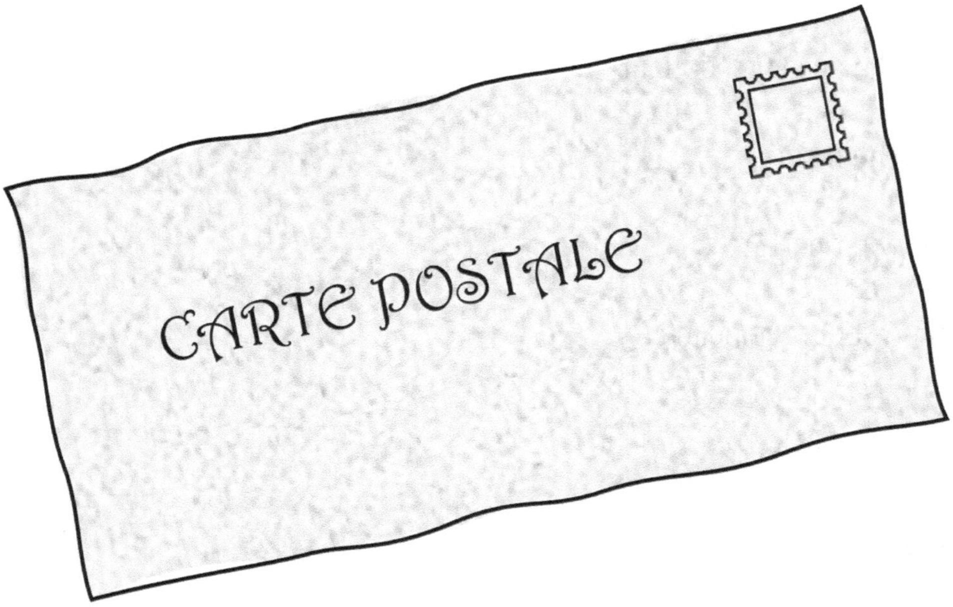

Therapy Targets

Activity 6: Finding smaller words from longer words

Instructions: How many little words can you make from each of the words below?

H O L I D A Y

C A M P I N G

C A M P E R V A N

Therapy Targets

Activity 7: Travel words

Instructions: Underline all the words related to travelling.

passport	rainbow	waiting area	aeroplane
border control	ferry	catapult	orange
desk	flight	journey	sight-seeing
passenger	daffodil	cruise	route
destination	luggage	voyage	garden
robin	excursion	check-in	tourist

Therapy Targets

Activity 8: Odd-one-out

Instructions: In each row, underline the word that does not belong with the others.

luggage	check-in	aeroplane	car
valley	passport	abroad	border control
trip	cathedral	excursion	sightseeing
cruise	ship	cabin	wing
taxi	train	coach	bus
suitcase	purse	luggage	rucksack
hiking	walking	rambling	camping

Therapy Targets

Activity 9(a): Categories

Instructions: How many words can you name for each category.

Holiday destinations	Clothing to pack for a summer holiday	Ways to travel

Therapy Targets

Activity 9(b): Categories – words provided

Instructions: Decide which word goes into each of the boxes.

train shorts Lake Garda aeroplane Paris

sunglasses Florida Cornwall ship New York

T-shirt sunhat bike Greece Disneyland

sandals coach swimsuit yacht London

Holiday destinations	Clothing to pack for a summer holiday	Ways to travel

Therapy Targets

Activity 10: What type of holiday?

Instructions: List as many different types of holiday as you can in the boxes below, e.g. sightseeing holiday.

Therapy Targets

Activity 11: The eco-friendly traveller

Instructions: Travel and tourism can have a detrimental impact on the environment. How could we make holidays more environmentally friendly?

Therapy Targets

Activity: Words of increasing length

Instructions: Read across each row. Say the words. Use the words in the third column to make a longer sentence.

The blank boxes at the bottom can be used for your own word sequences.

One syllable	Two syllables	Multisyllabic	Now say a complete sentence using the multisyllabic word or phrase
Plane	Aeroplane	Aeroplane landing	
Pass	Passport	Passport control	
Sand	Sandals	Silver sandals	
Lug	Luggage	Lost luggage	
Tick	Ticket	Train ticket	
Book	Booking	Hotel booking	

Therapy Targets

CHAPTER 9

THEME: TECHNOLOGY

CONTENTS				
ACTIVITY & PAGE NUMBER	**ACTIVITY**	**CLIENT GROUP**	**LEVEL**	**COMMENTS & SUGGESTIONS**
1(a) Page 102	Unscrambling crossword answers	Language or group	L1–L3	Different levels of task options given for different levels.
1(b) Pages 103–105	Crossword clues (with blank crossword and completed crossword)	Language or group	L1–L3	Blank crossword and completed crossword provided.
2 Pages 106–107	Computers word search	Language	L2–L3	Different levels of task options given for different levels.
3 Page 108	Ideas-web: computer	Language or group	L1–L2	
4 Page 109	Word-finder: Finding smaller words from a longer word	Language or group	L2–L3	Provide scrabble letters to make moving the letters around easier.
5 Pages 110–111	Word chain (with and without list of words)	Language or group	L2–L3	With help, this could be suitable for L1.
6 Page 112	Discussion points	Language, speech, group	L1–L3	
7 Pages 113–114	Technology through the ages	All	L1–L3	
8 Page 115	Satellite Wars!	All	L2–L3	
9 Page 116	Limerick	Speech, voice, fluency	L2–L3	

DOI: 10.4324/9781003177852-9

Activity 1(a): Unscrambling crossword answers

Instructions: Unscramble the words for the answers to the crossword given on page 3.

NB: the ones in *italics* are acronyms.

ACROSS:

3 S M E O U

4 N O

5 *D L E*

6 *B U S*

7 *M A R*

9 T P O R

DOWN:

1 O N C I

2 O A D E R B Y K

3 M O E M D

7 *R M O*

8 *P C U*

Therapy Targets

Activity 1(b): Crossword clues

Instructions: Read the clues below to complete the crossword on the following page.

TIP: If the person requires help to spell, write the words out for them to copy into the squares.

Across:

3 Used to move the curser

4 Before starting, turn the computer ...

5 Little light (acronym)

6 Commonly used computer socket (acronym)

7 Accessing memory can be variable (acronym)

9 Computer access terminal

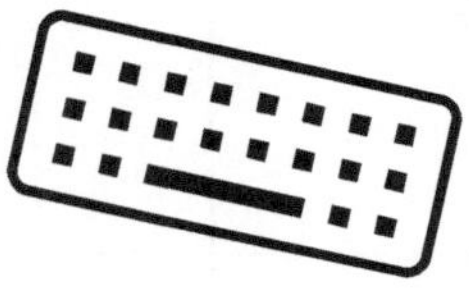

Down:

1 Small symbol to denote an app or program on a computer or phone, etc

2 Some people can touch-type on this

3 Device enabling computers to communicate via telephone lines

7 The constant memory of the computer (acronym)

8 Central processing unit (acronym)

Therapy Targets

Blank crossword for use with Activities 1 (a) and (b)

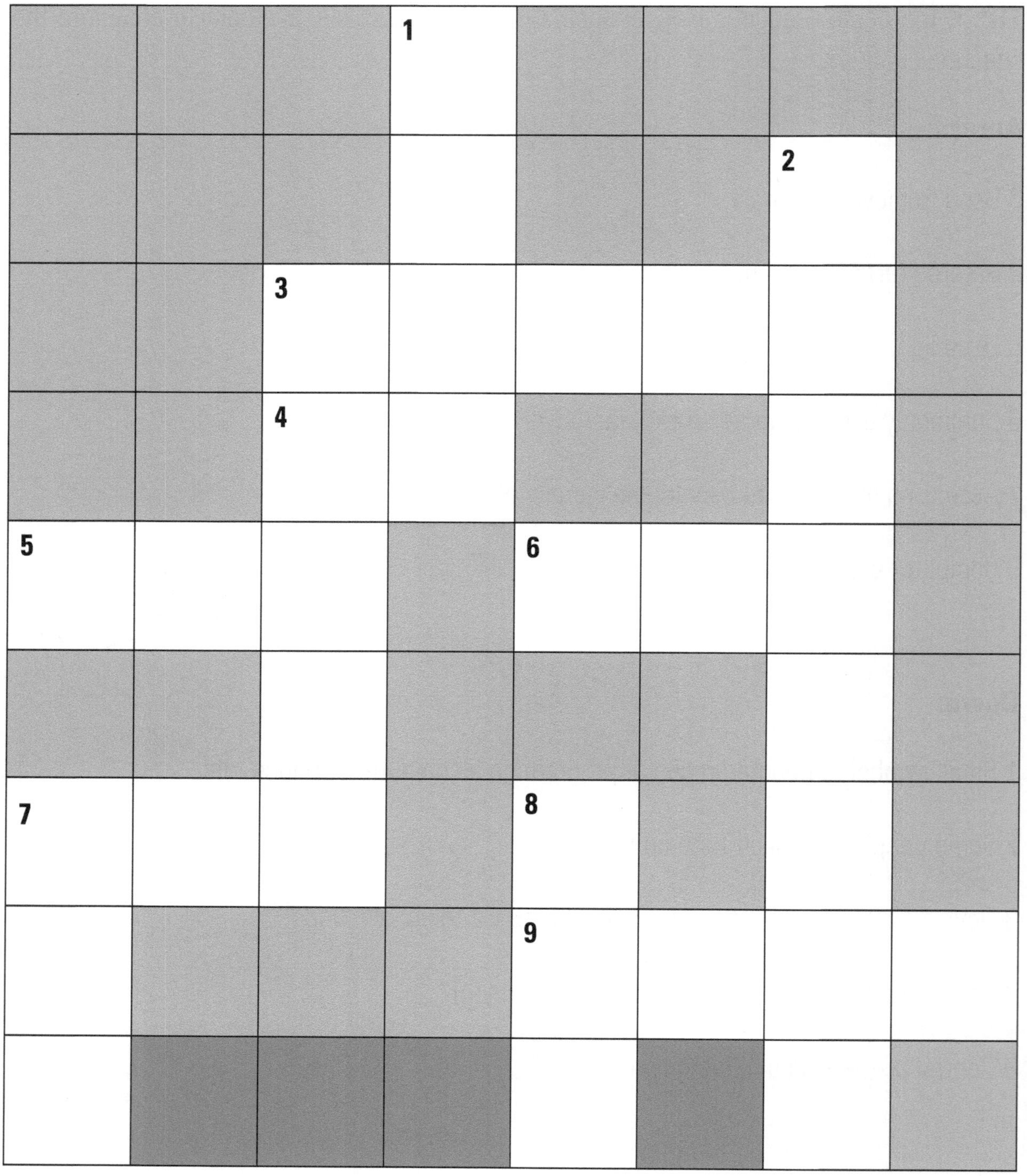

Completed crossword for use with Activities 1(a) and (b)

			1 I				
			C			2 K	
		3 M	O	U	S	E	
		4 O	N			Y	
5 L	E	D		6 U	S	B	
		E				O	
7 R	A	M		8 C		A	
O				9 P	0 O	R	T
M				U		D	

Activity 2: Computers word search

ALGORITHM

BROWSER

BOOT

BROADBAND

COMPUTER

GIGABYTE

FORMAT

FIREWALL

LAPTOP

MOUSE

NETWORK

POP

QWERTY

SCANNER

USERNAME

URL

USB

WEBSITE

ZIP

Tips for the word search exercise:

a) To make the task easier for your client, highlight the first letter or two.

b) To make it harder, do not provide a word list.

c) What other words, not related to computer words, can you find in the word search?

Therapy Targets

Activity 2: Computers word search

F	L	N	F	P	B	E	W	E	B	S	I	T	E	E	A
D	O	M	Y	N	E	T	W	O	R	K	D	I	K	M	P
S	R	R	O	P	B	V	C	P	O	P	Q	I	R	O	Y
A	T	L	M	E	S	B	E	Z	A	V	L	C	T	X	T
L	G	O	M	A	W	H	A	D	D	B	R	P	I	C	K
G	U	S	E	A	T	R	S	N	B	D	A	H	Q	K	F
O	I	Z	I	P	D	V	B	S	A	L	F	V	W	V	D
R	S	D	U	F	G	S	C	A	N	N	E	R	E	G	V
I	C	O	M	P	U	T	E	R	D	D	A	C	R	X	L
T	U	S	E	R	N	A	M	E	J	K	L	W	T	Y	L
H	Q	U	N	S	D	D	H	T	L	R	D	C	Y	F	A
M	M	G	D	E	E	U	T	S	U	A	D	C	M	T	W
F	G	I	G	A	B	Y	T	E	K	B	P	T	H	I	E
S	X	H	F	F	H	I	H	Y	M	F	X	O	C	D	R
N	Z	R	E	S	W	O	R	B	V	C	F	O	P	N	I
M	O	U	S	E	R	E	V	A	B	J	S	B	Q	L	F

Activity 3: Ideas-web: computer

Instructions: Thinking of the word computer, answer the questions in the ovals.

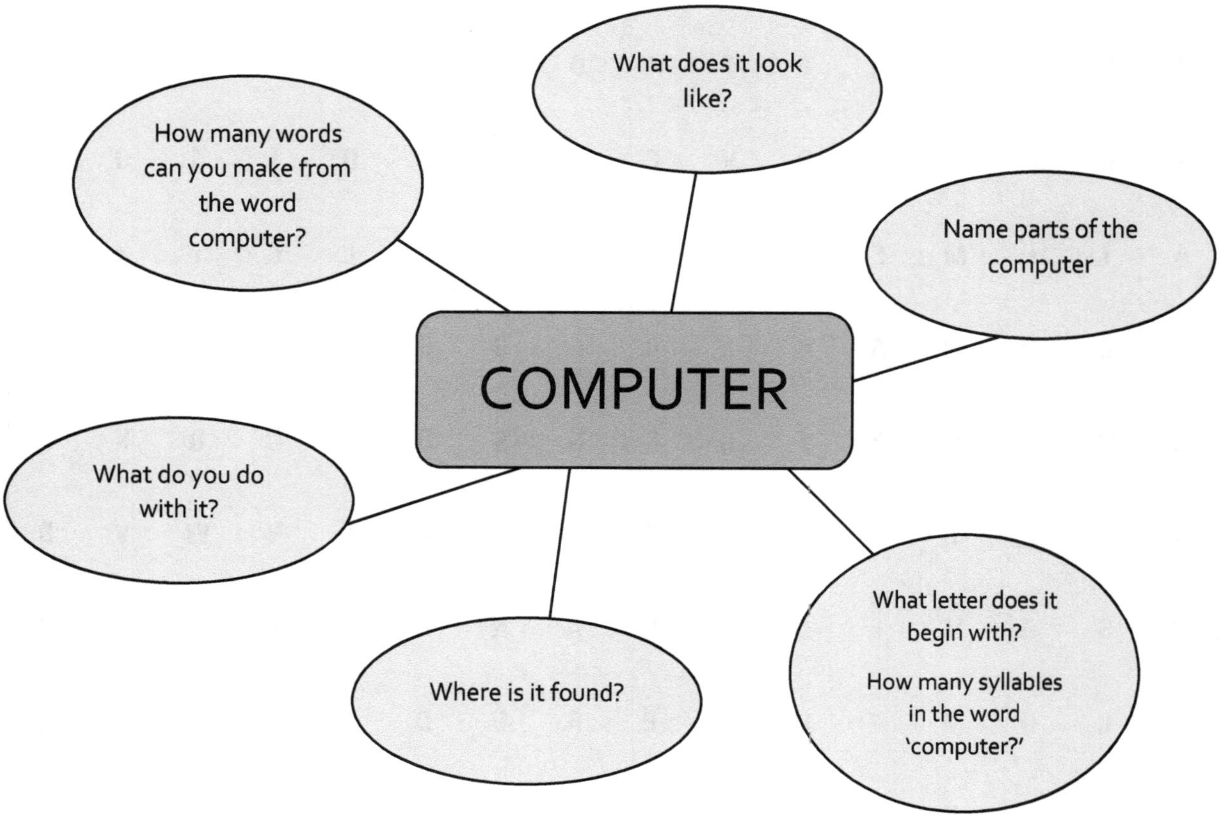

Replace the word in the middle with:

Mobile phone

Windfarm

Printer

Therapy Targets

Activity 4: Word-finder

Instructions: How many little words can you find in each of the words below?

FIREWALL

KEYBOARD

Therapy Targets

Activity 5(a): Word chain (with list of words)

Instructions: Use the words below to complete the word chain at the bottom of the page.

The last letter of the previous word becomes the first letter of the next word.

TABLET

RAM

TASKBAR

MODEM

PDF

MOUSE

LAPTOP

ETHERNET

MONITOR

EMAIL

ROM

FILE

Word chain: COMPUTE**R→R**A**M→M** _______

Therapy Targets

Activity 5(b): Word chain (without list of words)

Instructions: Using computer and technology terminology, create a chain of words.

The last letter of the previous word becomes the first letter of the next word.

COMPUTE**R**→**R**A**M**→**M** ________

Therapy Targets

Activity 6: Discussion topics

Instructions: Use the questions below to begin a discussion.

1) Has technology helped or hindered our lives? Explain your answer.

2) How has technology contributed to the environmental crisis?

3) How has technology changed in the last 20 years?

4) What do you think about wind farms and fields of solar panels?

5) Artificial Intelligence – friend or foe?

6) What is your favourite technological invention?

Therapy Targets

Activity 7(a): Technology through the ages

Instructions: Below are pictures of technological inventions. Arrange them into the order in which they were invented.

Either number the pictures or name them and write out your answers in the correct order.

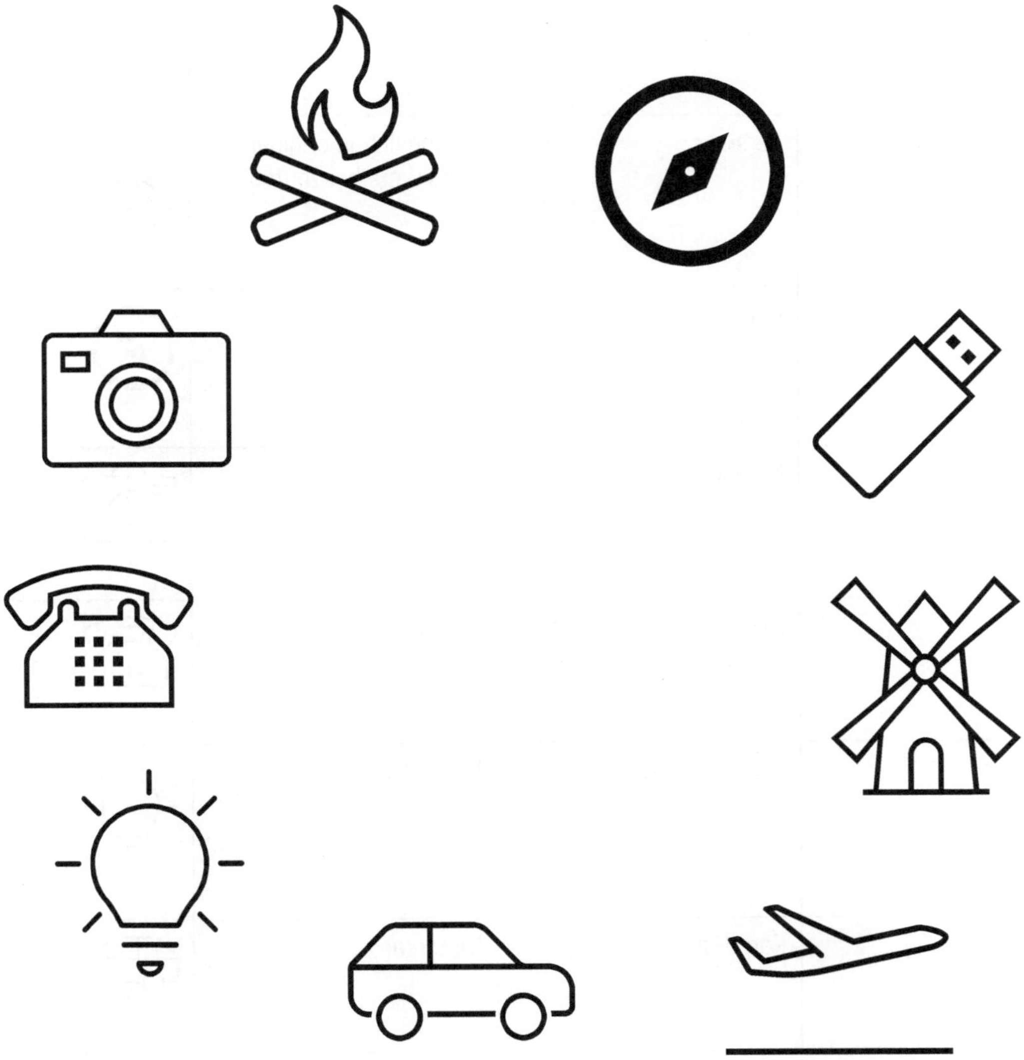

1) In which century were each of these invented?
2) Who invented them?

Therapy Targets

Activity 7(b): Technology through the ages – game ideas

Instructions: Use this information to make a quiz. Alternatively, cut out the pictures, dates and inventors and ask the client to match them up.

DATE	INVENTOR	INVENTION	
1 million years ago	Early man	Fire	
950	Persians	Windmill (the original ones were horizontal)	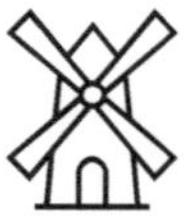
1044	Chinese	Compass	
1826 or 1827	Nicéphore Niépce	Camera	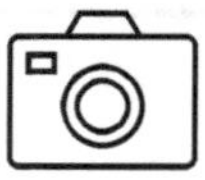
1876	Alexander Graham Bell	Telephone	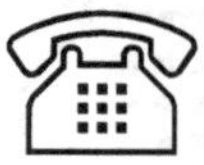
1879	Thomas Edison	Light bulb	
1885	Karl Benz	Motorcar	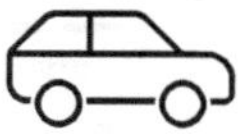
1903	Orville Wright	First air flight	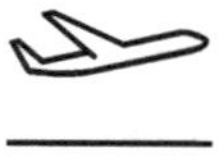
1990–1994	Amir Ban, Dov Moran, Oron Ogdan	USB flash drive	

Therapy Targets

Activity 8: Satellite Wars!

Instructions: Take it in turns to find the other person's satellite by giving a grid reference, for example: G4.

Who can find the most satellites?

One person uses this grid; the other person marks their satellites on a blank grid from the appendix (pen and paper grid wars).

H		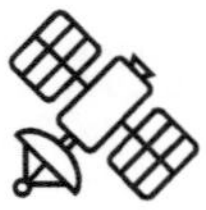						
G				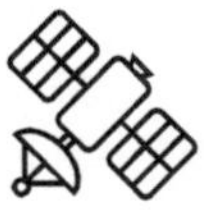			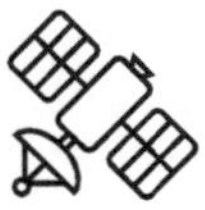	
F								
E								
D	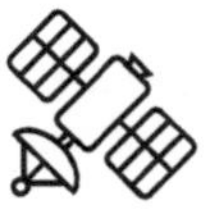							
C						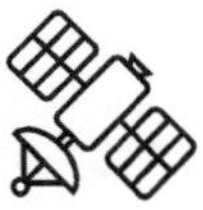		
B				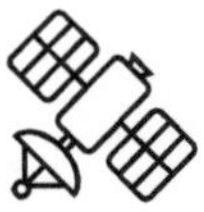				
A		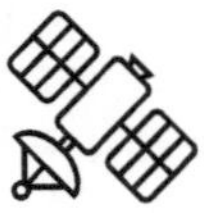						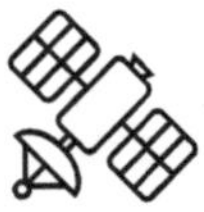
	1	2	3	4	5	6	7	8

Therapy Targets

Activity 9: Limerick

Instructions: See 'How to use this resource' chapter for ideas about how to use this limerick.

A mad man named Fin,
Had a windfarm within
A field that was part of his farm.
The wind once blew the fan right over a dam,
But at least thankful Fin came to no harm.

Neil Bonner (2021)

Therapy Targets

Activity: Words of increasing length

Instructions: Read across each row. Say the words. Use the words in the third column to make a longer sentence.

The blank boxes at the bottom can be used for your own word sequences.

One syllable	Two syllables	Multisyllabic	Now say a complete sentence using the multisyllabic word or phrase
In	Invent	Invention	
Wind	Windfarm	See the windfarm	
Screen	Flatscreen	Flatscreen television	
Mob	Mobile	Mobile phone number	
Why	Wifi	There's no wifi	
Mail	Email	Send an email	

Therapy Targets

CHAPTER 10

THEME: BIRDS

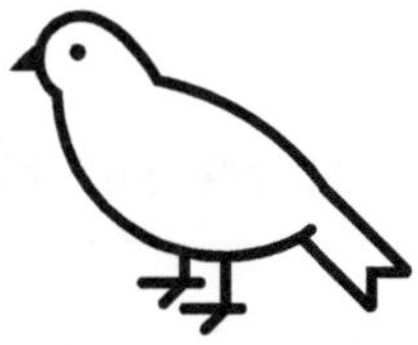

CONTENTS				
ACTIVITY & PAGE NUMBER	ACTIVITY	CLIENT GROUP	LEVEL	COMMENTS & SUGGESTIONS
1 Page 120	Proverbs & idioms	Language, speech, voice, fluency, group	L1–L3	Say aloud, complete the phrase or define the saying.
2 Page 121	Finding smaller words from a longer word	Language, groups	L2–L3	Good group activity.
3 Page 122	Comparisons	Language, speech, voice, fluency, group	L3 – some bird knowledge required	
4 Page 123	Word search 1 – bird names	Language	L1–L2	
5 Pages 124–125	Word search 2 – bird-related vocabulary	Language	L2–L3	
6 Page 126	Word definitions	Language, speech, voice, fluency, group	L3	
7 Page 127	Bird names – anagrams	Language	L1	
8(a) Page 128	Bird colour association	Language	L1–L2	
8(b) Page 129	Colour naming	Language	L2–L3	
9 Page 130	Find the verbs or read the passage aloud	Language (reading), speech, voice, fluency	L2–L3	

DOI: 10.4324/9781003177852-10

Activity 1: Proverbs and idioms

Instructions: Read these proverbs and idioms aloud. Or, the therapist can read the first part aloud for the client to complete.

Free as a bird.

Like a duck to water.

Like water off a duck's back.

A bird in the hand is worth two in the bush.

Birds of a feather flock together.

The early bird catches the worm.

As graceful as a swan.

Take someone under your wing.

Proud as a peacock.

As the crow flies.

Don't count your chickens until they are hatched.

Feather your nest.

Happy as a lark.

Therapy Targets

Activity 2: Finding smaller words from a longer word

Instructions: How many little words can you find in the word below?

As an extra challenge, arrange them into alphabetical order.

BINOCULARS

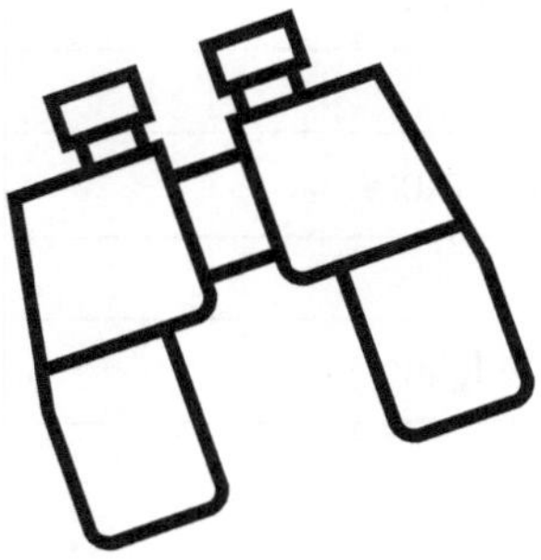

Therapy Targets

Activity 3: Comparisons

Instructions: Describe the similarities and differences between the terms below.

Birdwatcher	Twitcher
Binoculars	Telescope
Blue tit	Bearded tit
Waders	Shorebirds
Duck	Mallard
Resident (or sedentary)	Migratory
Hatchling	Fledgling

Therapy Targets

Activity 4: Word search 1

Instructions: Find the names of these birds in the letter grid below:

THRUSH ROBIN SPARROW WREN LARK DUCK

P	T	H	R	U	S	H	R
S	P	A	R	R	O	W	O
K	A	R	N	O	U	M	B
K	L	E	Z	D	W	S	I
A	R	H	N	U	C	R	N
W	J	A	X	C	I	V	B
Y	P	R	L	K	E	F	G

Therapy Targets

Activity 5(a): Word search 2

Instructions: Find bird-related words in the letter grid below.

Either see how many you can find without the list, or use the word list in Activity 5(b) to find the words.

U	I	B	B	I	N	O	C	U	L	A	R	S	G	B	U
Z	F	E	E	D	F	K	C	W	I	E	B	M	L	I	F
M	A	O	J	K	A	E	B	N	V	E	D	K	M	R	U
I	S	A	R	X	O	D	N	S	U	T	L	C	S	D	I
G	L	E	X	N	E	P	E	L	A	G	I	C	R	W	E
R	V	E	D	L	I	A	J	I	O	T	F	T	E	A	M
A	S	Q	U	E	L	T	C	A	M	V	U	N	I	T	E
T	O	E	B	C	N	R	H	S	T	W	E	A	D	C	N
I	S	H	I	S	R	T	Y	O	L	E	G	R	V	H	U
O	U	E	F	E	A	N	A	M	L	G	C	G	K	E	N
N	E	T	N	S	U	H	R	R	E	O	B	A	M	R	T
R	E	W	M	I	M	X	Q	U	Y	S	G	V	L	I	O
K	I	R	E	L	B	R	A	W	R	S	E	Y	N	P	R

Therapy Targets

Activity 5(b): Word search 2 (words provided)

Instructions: Find the bird-related words in the letter grid in Activity 5(a).

The words might be up, down, diagonal, and backwards.

ORNITHOLOGY

BIRDWATCHER

WARBLER

BINOCULARS

PELAGIC

MIGRATION

SEDENTARY

NEST

BEAK

VAGRANT

FEED

EGG

Therapy Targets

Activity 6: Word definitions

Instructions: Define the words below.

ORNITHOLOGY

BIRDWATCHER

WARBLER

BINOCULARS

PELAGIC

MIGRATION

SEDENTARY

NEST

BEAK

VAGRANT

FEED

EGG

Therapy Targets

Activity 7: Bird names – anagrams

Instructions: Unscramble these letters for common bird names.

3-letter words:

T T I

Y J A

W L O

M U E

N H E

4-letter words:

L U L G

N W E R

E V O D

C U K D

B I S I

K W I I

N S W A

K L A R

Therapy Targets

Activity 8(a): Bird colour association

Instructions: Match the colour associated with each bird.

ROBIN	BROWN
WREN	GREY
BLACKBIRD	BLUE
KINGFISHER	WHITE
SWAN	RED
DOVE	BLACK

Therapy Targets

Activity 8(b): Colour naming

Instructions: What colours do you associate with each bird?

ROBIN

MAGPIE

WREN

WOODPECKER

BLACKBIRD

SISKIN

FLAMINGO

DOVE

SWAN

PEACOCK

Therapy Targets

Activity 9: Find the verbs

Instructions: Underline the verbs in the passage below.

Identifying different birds can be a tricky business. The novice might be confused by similarities between some birds. For example, do you know your coal tit from your blue tit? Identifying different species is often more challenging because the birds flit about or may be some distance away. However, considering a few basic points can help you to spot your bullfinch from your brambling.

As well as learning a few basic markings, it is possible to identify a bird based on what time of year it is seen, where it is feeding and its song. For example, a fieldfare is a winter visitor to Britain, feeds on berries in the hedgerow and has a chattery type of song. Its lookalike, the song thrush, is resident in Britain throughout the year, feeds on snails and has a loud, distinctive song marked by a repetition of two or three 'phrases'.

In order to watch birds, a quiet disposition, patience, and a good pair of binoculars come in extremely useful!

Therapy Targets

Activity: Words of increasing length

Instructions: Read across each row. Say the words. Use the words in the third column to make a longer sentence.

The blank boxes at the bottom can be used for your own word sequences.

One syllable	Two syllables	Multisyllabic	Now say a complete sentence using the multisyllabic word or phrase
Fledge	Fledgling	Fledgling birds	
Black	Blackbird	Blackbird's nest	
Fly	Flying	Flying away	
Peck	Pecking	Pecking order	
Rob	Robin	Robin redbreast	
Feed	Feeding	Feeding the young	

Therapy Targets

CHAPTER 11

THEME: GARDENING

CONTENTS				
ACTIVITY & PAGE NUMBER	**ACTIVITY**	**CLIENT GROUP**	**LEVEL**	**COMMENTS & SUGGESTIONS**
1 Page 134	Gardening tools – anagrams	Language, groups	L2–L3	
2 Page 135	Naming gardening tools	Language, speech, voice, fluency, group	L1–L3	People at L1 might need some help.
3 Page 136	Word generator	Language, groups	L2–L3	L1 – use scrabble letters to make anagrams from the letters.
4 Page 137	Garden-themed idioms	Language, speech, voice, fluency, group	L2–L3	
5(a) Page 138	Garden tools and their jobs	Language	L1	
5(b) Page 139	Garden tools and their jobs	Language, speech, voice, fluency, group	L2–L3	
6 Page 140	Naming flowers	Language, speech, voice, fluency, group	L2–L3	L1 – provide the names of flowers and ask the person to allocate to the right category.
7 Page 141	Word ladder	Language	L2	
8(a)–8(c) Pages 142–144	Sentence sequencing	Language, speech, voice, fluency, group	L2–L3	Cut out the sentences and ask the person to arrange them into order.
9 Page 145	Written word to picture matching	Language	L1	Write out the words for the person to match to the pictures.

DOI: 10.4324/9781003177852-11

Activity 1: Anagrams – naming gardening tools

Instructions: Unscramble the anagrams to name some tools.

K R O F

E H O

E D S P A

H E A S R S

T E C S U R S A E

K R E A

H E L R E A B R O W W

Therapy Targets

Activity 2: Naming gardening tools

Instructions: How many gardening tools can you name?

TIP: Look through a gardening magazine or book to give you some ideas.

Therapy Targets

Activity 3: Word generator

Instructions: Using the letters in the petals, how many words can you make using three letters or more? They do not have to be words related to gardening.

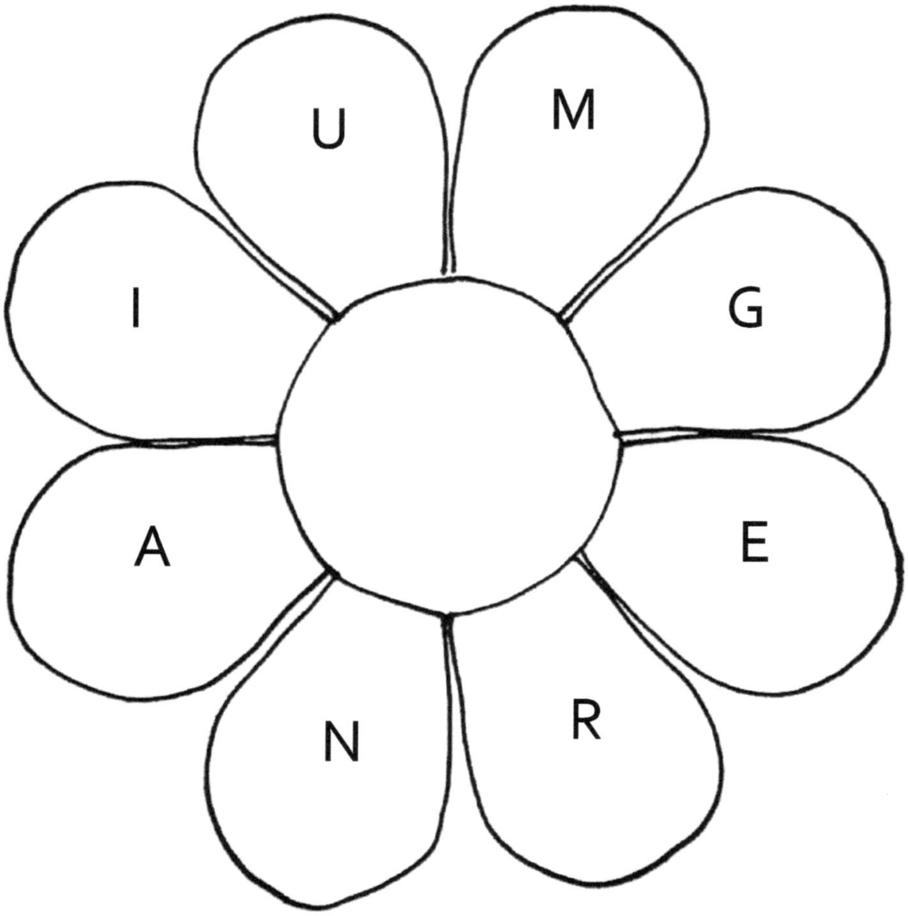

Therapy Targets

Activity 4: Garden-themed idioms

Instructions: Say the following idioms aloud.

Everything in the garden is rosy.

Common or garden variety.

Make hay whilst the sun shines.

You've been led down the garden path.

She's a shrinking violet.

Stop beating about the bush.

Money doesn't grow on trees.

It's a tough row to hoe.

He calls a spade a spade.

Give it some welly!

Don't make a mountain out of a molehill.

Can you explain what these idioms mean?

Therapy Targets

Activity 5(a): Garden tools and their jobs

Instructions: Look at the gardening jobs in the box below. Match the jobs with the tools in the list. Write it next to the tool or say it aloud.

making holes for seeds	digging	cutting grass	collecting leaves	cutting edges of flower beds	moving heavy items	pruning	watering the tubs

Lawnmower →

Rake →

Secateurs →

Dibber →

Edge cutter →

Spade →

Wheelbarrow →

Watering can →

Therapy Targets

Activity 5(b): Garden tools and their jobs

Instructions: What do you use these tools for in the garden?

Hoe →

Lawnmower →

Rake →

Secateurs →

Dibber →

Edge cutter →

Spade →

Wheelbarrow →

Watering can →

1) Can you write your answers in full sentences?
   E.g. 'Hoe' – a hoe is used for weeding.
2) Which is your favourite gardening job?
3) Which is your least favourite gardening job?

Therapy Targets

Activity 6: Naming flowers

Instructions: Name some flowers according to the prompts.

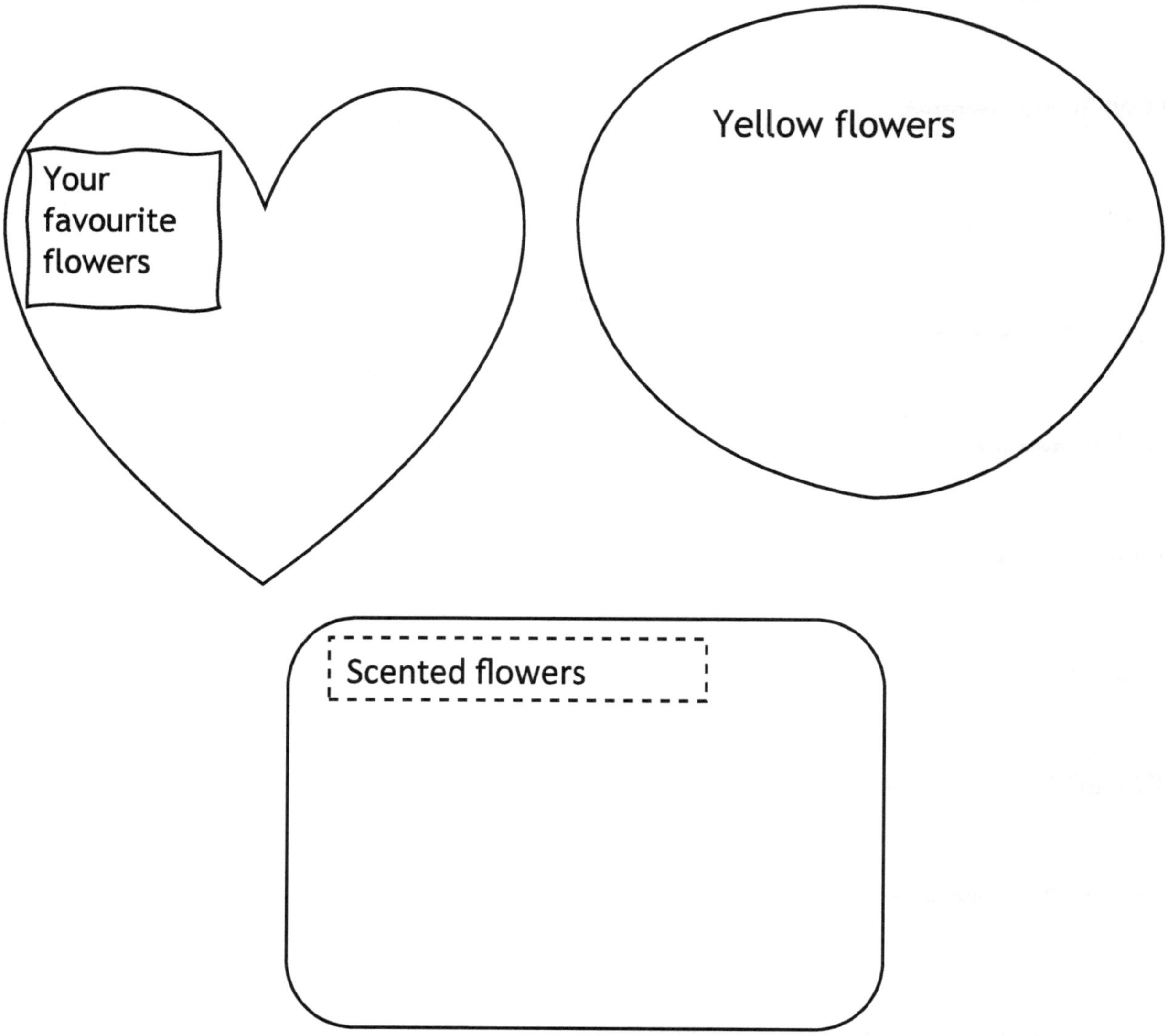

Therapy Targets

Activity 7: Word ladder

Instructions: Change one letter at a time to change the word.

Change any letter each time. The word does not have to relate to gardening.

W	E	E	D

Therapy Targets

Activity 8(a): Sentence sequencing

Instructions: Arrange the sentences into the correct order to describe how to do the following gardening task.

Sowing seeds outside:

Sprinkle seeds into the row.

Water the row.

Select the seeds.

Cover the seeds.

Prepare the ground.

Label the row of seeds.

Make a shallow row.

Therapy Targets

Activity 8(b): Sentence sequencing

Instructions: Arrange the sentences into the correct order to describe how to do the following gardening task.

Planting out a potted plant:

Firm the soil around the plant.

Water the hole.

Gently loosen the roots.

Dig a hole.

Put some compost in the bottom of the hole.

Water the plant an hour before transplanting.

Water the newly transplanted plant.

Take the plant out of the pot.

Place the plant roots into the hole.

Fill the rest of the hole with compost.

Therapy Targets

Activity 8(c): Sentence sequencing

Instructions: Arrange the sentences into the correct order to describe how to do the following gardening task.

Weeding:

Continue digging out all the weeds.

Rake over the weeded area to level out the soil.

Shake the soil off the root ball.

Put your gardening tools away.

Dig up a weed.

Find your trug basket or bucket.

Decide where to start weeding.

Put the weeds into your trug basket or bucket.

Fetch your garden rake and fork.

Empty the trug basket into the bin or compost.

Therapy Targets

Activity 9: Written word to picture matching

Instructions: Write the name next to the picture.

seedling	trowel & fork	butterfly	seeds
bird	watering can	flower	wheelbarrow

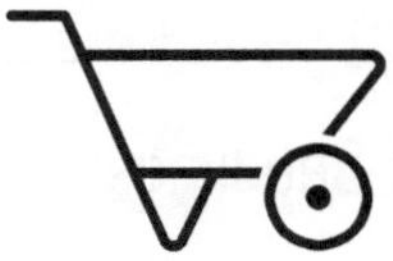

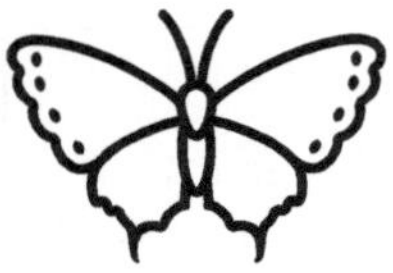

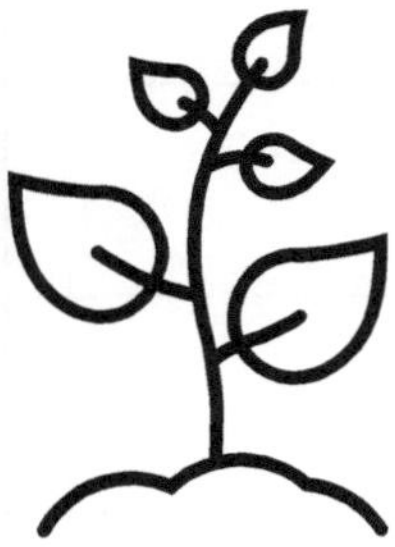

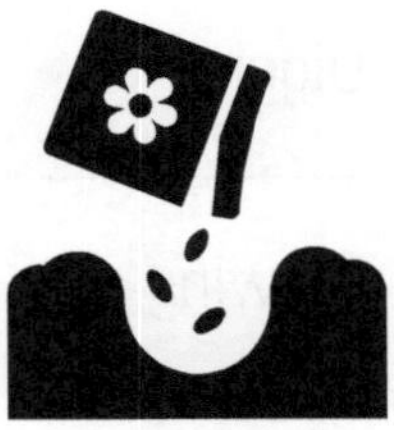

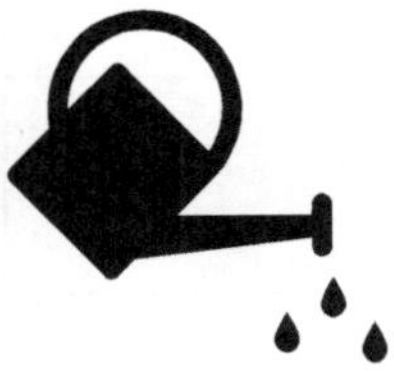

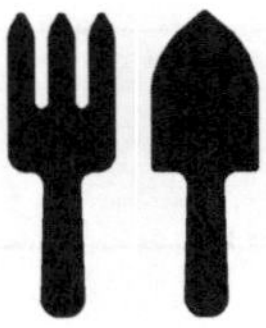

Therapy Targets

Activity: Words of increasing length

Instructions: Read across each row. Say the words. Use the words in the third column to make a longer sentence.

The blank boxes at the bottom can be used for your own word sequences.

One syllable	Two syllables	Multisyllabic	Now say a complete sentence using the multisyllabic word or phrase
Seed	Seedlings	Thin out the seedlings	
Grow	Growing	Growing vegetables	
Plant	Planting	Planting out the shrubs	
Pot	Plant pot	Plant pot stand	
Dig	Digging	Digging the garden	
Mow	Mowing	Mowing the lawn	

Therapy Targets

THEME: GOLF

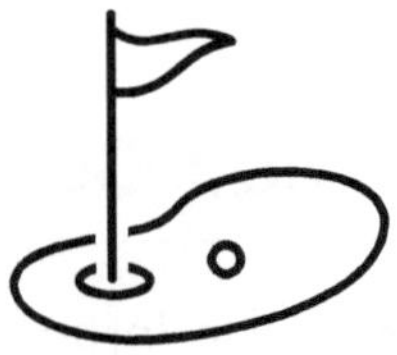

CONTENTS

DOI: 10.4324/9781003177852-12

Activity 1(a): Golfing equipment

Instructions: Underline the terms below that relate to golf.

club	ball	dog	coffee
bat	tees	net	ball marker
pram	buggy	wallet	bag
button	towel	rangefinder	irons
golden retriever	cheese	grass	ball retriever
club headcover	crayon	divot	cart
wedges	triangles	Land Rover	ball washer

What other words come to mind when you think about golf?

Therapy Targets

Activity 1(b): Golfing equipment

Instructions: Make a list of golfing equipment.

TIP: Look through a golfing magazine to help find words.

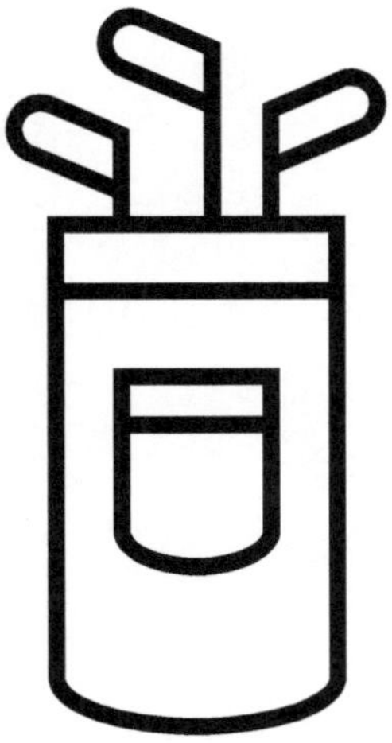

Therapy Targets

Activity 1(c): Golfing equipment and clothing memory game

Instructions: This is like the game, 'I went to market to buy...'. This time say, 'I went golfing and forgot to take my...'

TIP: Use mimes to remind each other of the items on the list.

To start you off:

"I went golfing and forgot to take my tee"
Next person says, "I went golfing and forgot to take my tee and my......"

Therapy Targets

Activity 2: Explaining the rules

Instructions: Write down or explain the rules of golf. Imagine the person you are talking to has never played a game of golf before.

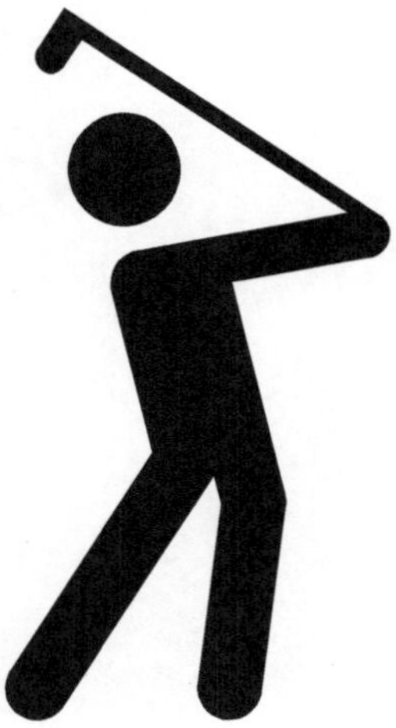

Therapy Targets

Activity 3: Golfing phrases

Instructions: Practise saying these golfing words and phrases.

That's a birdie.

What's your handicap?

In the leather.

That's out of bounds.

We're at the turn.

What a whiff!

I'm in the zone today.

Oh no! What a flub!

That was a duff shot, mate.

He's a bit of a duffer.

She's part of the dawn patrol.

Let's head over to the dance floor.

You're going to need to do a backhander.

Time for tee-off.

Therapy Targets

Activity 4: Board game – places on the golf course

Instructions: Get your dice and counters. Go round the golf course, saying the names of the places on the course when you land on them. If you roll a 5 or a 6, there are other people on the course – you have to stay put until your next turn!

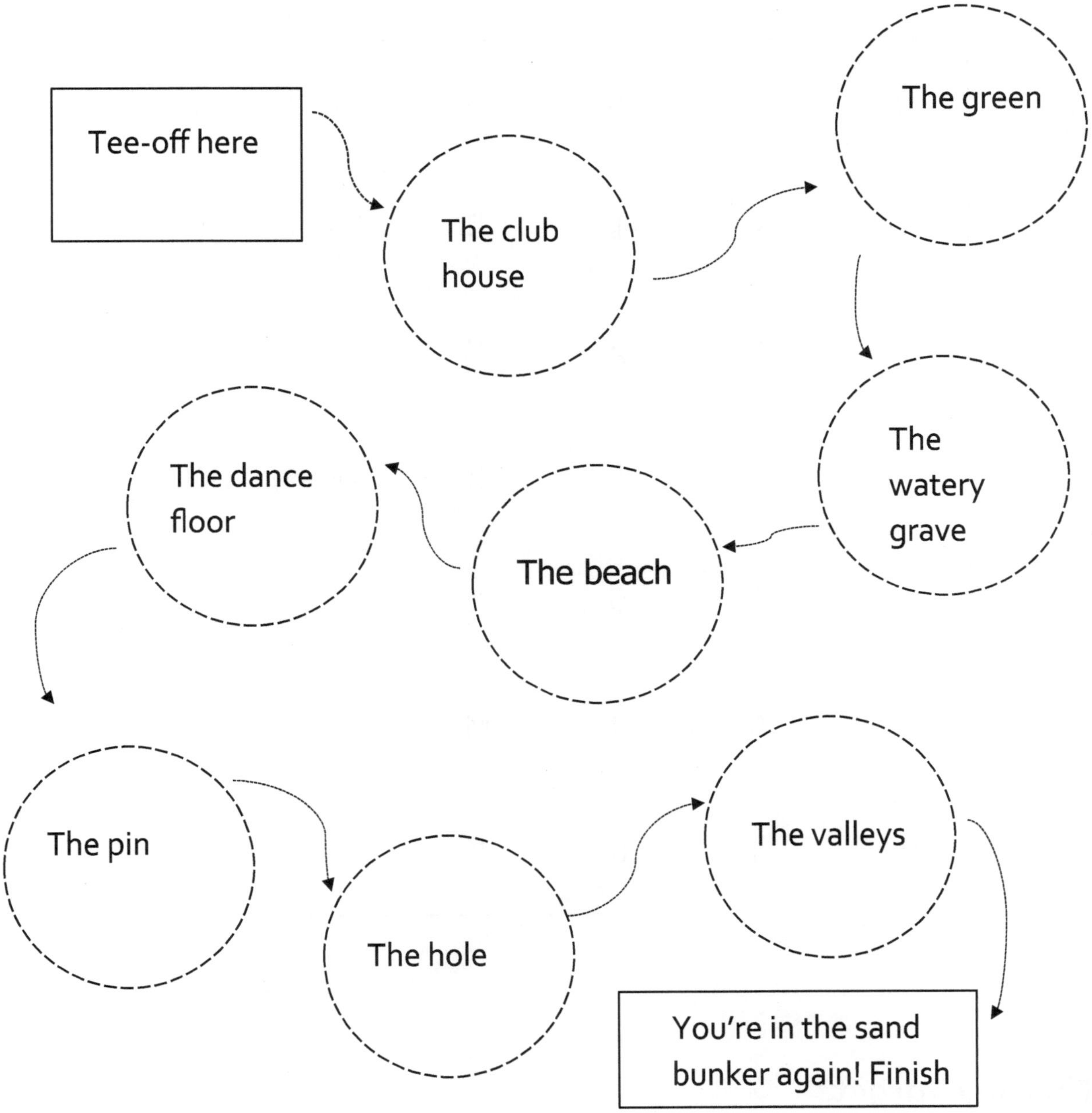

Therapy Targets

Activity 5: Golf word search

Instructions: Find the words below in the letter grid.

golf	player	bag	club	tee

F	H	G	O	L	F
Z	A	L	D	W	M
P	L	A	Y	E	R
M	G	C	R	B	N
G	B	Q	X	U	T
K	A	J	M	L	E
E	O	B	P	C	E

Therapy Targets

Activity 6: Know your clubs from your irons

Instruction: Draw a line between the ovals to link up the golfclub name with its description.

The driver	A combination of the woods and the irons
The fairway	Used for tee shots on short holes
The irons	Knocking the ball into the hole
The hybrids	Used for long shots – smaller clubhead
The putter	Used for long shots – larger 'face'

Therapy Targets

Activity 7(a): Golf courses and locations

Instructions: Match the golf course to the country. Write your answer in the box next to the golf course. Table of answers provided on page 158.

St. Andrews		Australia
Royal County Down		Scotland
Cypress Point		Ireland
Kingston Heath		Wales
Royal Porthcawl		USA
Royal St. George's		Northern Ireland
Ballybunion		Australia
Trump Turnberry		England
Shinnecock Hills		Scotland
Sunningdale		Wales
Royal Durnoch		England
Royal Melbourne		USA
Royal St. David's		Australia
Kingston Heath		Scotland

Therapy Targets

Activity 7(b): Golf courses and locations

Instructions: Cut out the table of courses and their countries on page 158. These 'cards' can be used in a number of ways:

1) Ask the client to match them up.
2) Play a memory game. Place all the 'cards' face down. Take it in turns to turn over two 'cards'. Try to find a matching course and location. Who can find the most pairs?
3) Photocopy the page twice. Play the memory game, matching only the golf courses or only the countries.
4) Put numbers on the back of the location cards and place them face down.
   Place the courses cards face up.
   Roll a dice. Pick up the card corresponding to the number and match the location to the course.
   As locations are found, replace with the remaining locations (do not forget to add the right number).
5) The therapist can name the location, and the client names the golf course found there.

Therapy Targets

Table of answers for Activities 7(a) and 7(b)

St. Andrews	Scotland
Royal County Down	Northern Ireland
Cypress Point	USA
Kingston Heath	Australia
Royal Porthcawl	Wales
Royal St. George's	England
Ballybunion	Ireland
Trump Turnberry	Scotland
Shinnecock Hills	USA
Sunningdale	England
Kingston Heath	Australia
Royal Durnoch	Scotland
Royal Melbourne	Australia
Royal St. David's	Wales

Therapy Targets

Activity 8(a): Word definitions – golfing terms

Instructions: Define these golfing terms. Table of answers provided on page 162.

Birdie

Tee-off

Handicap

Irons

Bunker

Hole out

Divot

Double Bogey

Therapy Targets

Activity 8(b): Word definitions – golfing terms

Instructions: Read the definition and name it. Alternatively, write the term in the box next to it. Table of answers provided on page 162.

	A score of one under the par for a hole.
	Start of the game.
	A scoring system that takes into account the ability of the golfer before they are awarded a score.
	A type of golf club.
	An area on the course emptied of turf and prepared as a hazard by filling it with sand or a similar substance. The lip of a bunker that is not covered in grass is also considered part of the bunker. Specific rules apply when playing from bunkers that are different to normal play.
	To continue playing the hole until the ball enters the hole.
	The turf removed from the ground during a golf shot; it usually creates a hole.
	A score of two over the par for the hole

Therapy Targets

Activity 8(c): Word definition – golfing terms

Instructions: Cut out the terms and definitions in the table below. Mix them up, then ask the person to match them up again. Table of answers provided on page 162.

Birdie	A score of one under the par for a hole.
Tee-off	Start of the game.
Handicap	A scoring system that takes into account the ability of the golfer before they are awarded a score.
Irons	A type of golf club.
Bunker	An area on the course emptied of turf and prepared as a hazard by filling it with sand or a similar substance. The lip of a bunker that is not covered in grass is also considered part of the bunker. Specific rules apply when playing from bunkers that are different to normal play.
Hole out	To continue playing the hole until the ball enters the hole.
Divot	The turf removed from the ground during a golf shot; it usually creates a hole.
Double Bogey	A score of two over the par for the hole.

Table of answers for Activities 8(a)–8(c)

Birdie	A score of one under the par for a hole.
Tee-off	Start of the game.
Handicap	A scoring system that takes into account the ability of the golfer before they are awarded a score.
Irons	A type of golf club.
Bunker	An area on the course emptied of turf and prepared as a hazard by filling it with sand or a similar substance. The lip of a bunker that is not covered in grass is also considered part of the bunker. Specific rules apply when playing from bunkers that are different to normal play.
Hole out	To continue playing the hole until the ball enters the hole.
Divot	The turf removed from the ground during a golf shot; it usually creates a hole.
Double Bogey	A score of two over the par for the hole.

Activity: Words of increasing length

Instructions: Read across each row. Say the words. Use the words in the third column to make a longer sentence.

The blank boxes at the bottom can be used for your own word sequences.

One syllable	Two syllables	Multisyllabic	Now say a complete sentence using the multisyllabic word or phrase
Golf	Golfing	Golfing tournament	
Golf	Golfclub	Golfclub bag	
Bird	Birdie	That's a birdie	
Put	Putting	Putting the ball	
Drive	Driver	Use the driver	
Club	Clubhouse	Go to the clubhouse	

Therapy Targets

CHAPTER 13

THEME: FOOD & DRINK

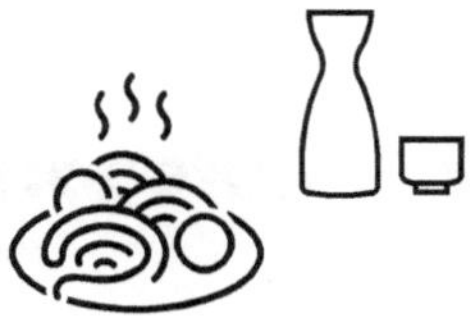

CONTENTS				
ACTIVITY & PAGE NUMBER	**ACTIVITY**	**CLIENT GROUP**	**LEVEL**	**COMMENTS & SUGGESTIONS**
1 Page 166	Categorising fruit and vegetables	Language, group	L1	Could be adapted into a speech exercise (single word or simple sentences).
2 Page 167	Word recall	All		Provide words for L1 clients to sort into category per letter.
3(a) Page 168	Ingredients – vegetable balti	All	L1–L3	
3(b) Page 169	Ingredients – chicken stir fry	All	L1–L3	
3(c) Page 170	Ingredients – beef casserole	All	L1–L3	
4 Page 171	Planning and sequencing	All	L2–L3	Write out the steps to be put into order for L1 clients.
5(a)–(d) Pages 172–175	Food spellings	Language (written)	L1 for 5(a) & (b) L2 for 5(c) & (d)	
6 Page 176-177	Food quiz	All	L1–L3	For L1, provide pictures or written answers for the client to point to.
7(a)–7(b) Pages 178–179	Synonyms	Language, group		7(a) geared to L1–L2 & 7(b) geared to L3.
8 Page 180	Favourite food and drink	All	L1–L3	Provide pictures or words to help L1 clients.

DOI: 10.4324/9781003177852-13

Activity 1: Categorising fruit and vegetables

Instructions: Look at the groceries in the box below. Decide whether they are fruit or a vegetable and write their name in the corresponding column.

pear	carrot	apple	pineapple	swede	parsnip
cabbage	tomato	yam	beetroot	okra	mango
mushroom	lychees	onion	banana	potato	raspberry
water chestnuts	peas	leeks	courgette or zucchini	strawberry	pak choi

VEGETABLE	FRUIT

Therapy Targets

Activity 2: Word recall

Instructions: List foods that begin with the given letter.

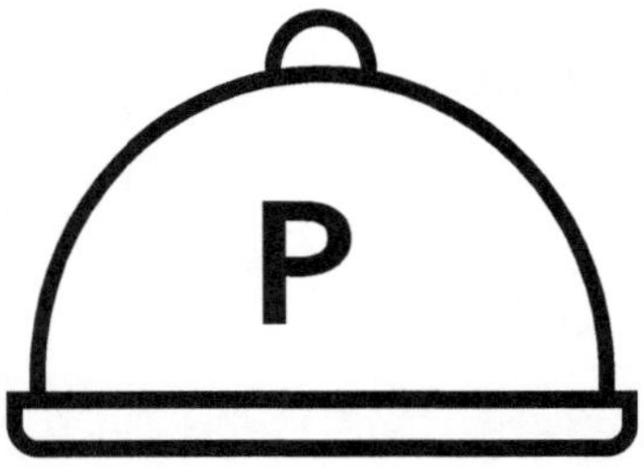

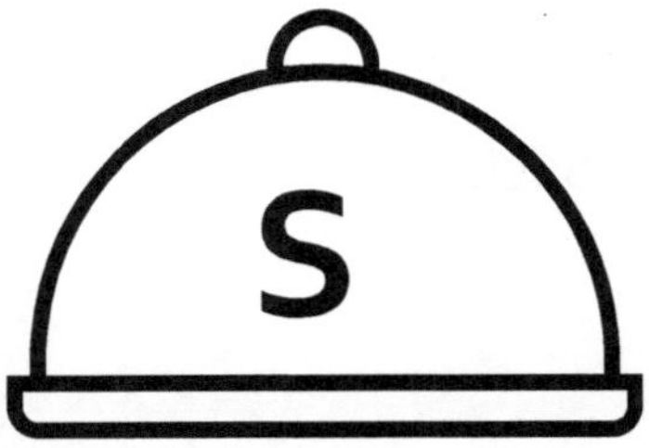

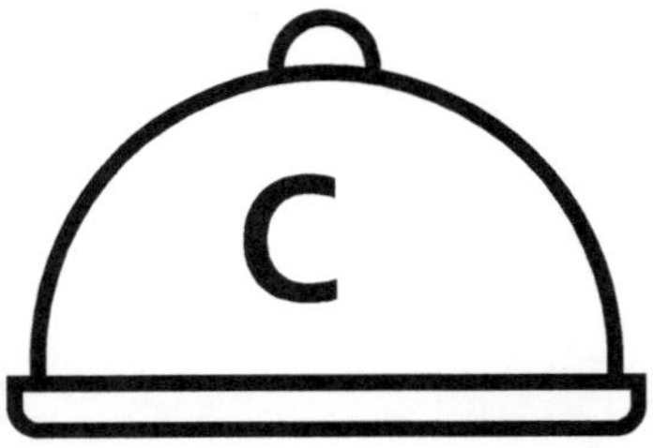

Can you think of one drink beginning with each of the letters?

Therapy Targets

Activity 3(a): Ingredients – vegetable balti

Instructions: Underline the ingredients you need to make a vegetable balti.

pasta	carrots	onion	water
cumin	tomatoes	pear	potato
avocado	cauliflower	chicken	turmeric
ginger	soy sauce	garam masala	apple
garlic	coriander	water chestnuts	
paprika	sugar	bread sweetcorn	

Therapy Targets

Activity 3(b): Ingredients – chicken stir fry

Instructions: Underline the ingredients you need to make a chicken stir fry.

onion	pasta	carrots	water
peas	soy sauce	pear	potato
avocado	red pepper	chicken	rice
ginger	sesame oil	beef	lavender
garlic	bay leaf	water chestnuts	
broccoli	sugar	bread	sweetcorn

Therapy Targets

Activity 3(c): Ingredients – beef casserole

Instructions: Underline the ingredients you need to make a beef casserole.

bay leaf	celery	carrots	milk
peas	mayonnaise	beef stock	potato
avocado	red pepper	chicken	rice
ginger	orange	beef	honey
garlic	beansprouts	beer	leeks
broccoli	mixed herbs	bread	onion

Therapy Targets

Activity 4: Planning and sequencing

Instructions: Describe how you would make each of the following. Give as much detail as possible.

Example: making a cup of tea.

1) fill the kettle with water
2) switch the kettle on and wait for it to boil
3) find a mug
4) put the teabag into the mug
5) fetch a teaspoon
6) When the kettle has boiled, pour the water into the mug
7) Stir the teabag then remove it
8) get the milk and pour some into the mug

Now write or say how you would make these food and drinks:

a) a cup of coffee
b) a jam sandwich
c) a pint of shandy
d) cheese on toast
e) an egg mayonnaise sandwich
f) a cake
g) a vegetable balti
h) a chicken stir fry
i) a beef casserole

Therapy Targets

Activity 5(a): Food spellings (3-letter words)

Instructions: Complete the spellings of food and drink. Choose one of the letters in brackets to complete the word.

eg_ (g j)

oi_ (l m)

pi_ (e a)

ha_ (p m)

pe_ (a c) 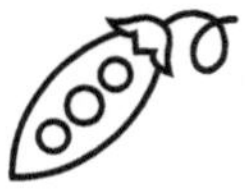

ya_ (k m)

_ut (k n) 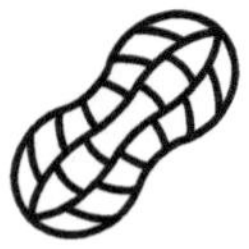

ja_ (a m)

_od (c h) 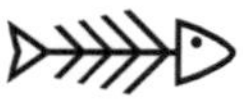

Therapy Targets

Activity 5(b): Food spellings (4-letter words)

Instructions: Complete the spellings. Choose one of the letters in brackets to complete the word.

_alt (t s)

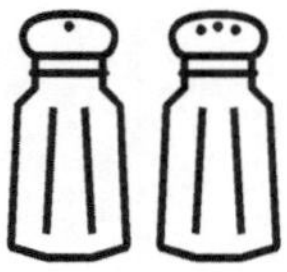

ri_e (c z)

p_as (l e)

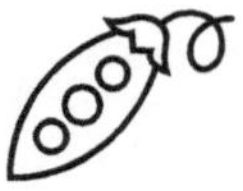

fis_ (c h)

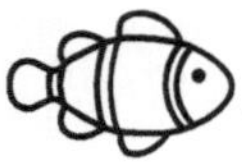

okr_ (a h)

_ilk (n m)

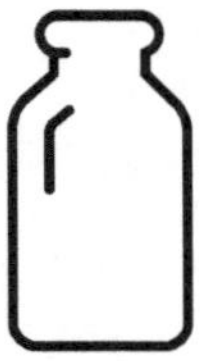

tac_ (u o)

p_ar (e l)

_ake (l c)

Therapy Targets

Activity 5(c): Food spellings (5-letter words)

Instructions: Complete the spellings.

TIP: Helper can provide a couple of written letter options if required.

ap_le 

patt_

hon_y 

B_lti

pea_h 

curr_

piz_a 

sals_

brea_ 

_asta

le_on 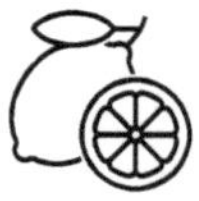

Therapy Targets

Activity 5(d): Food spellings (6-letter words)

Instructions: Complete the spellings.

TIP: Helper can provide a couple of written letter options if required.

chi_li 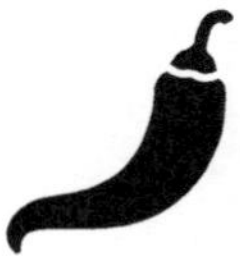

gar_ic

pe_per

ora_ge 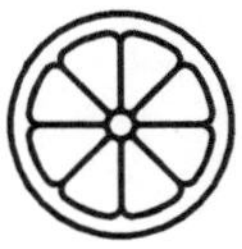

ca_rot

muf_in 

_ogurt

c_eese 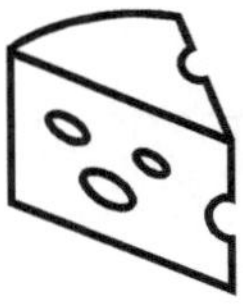

to_ato

salmo_ 

pota_o

gra_es 

Therapy Targets

Activity 6: Food quiz

Instructions: The quiz can be presented verbally or given to the person to write their answers.

The answers are provided on the following page.

1) Finish the film title: Cloudy with a Chance of ... .
2) According to the Office for National Statistics, in 2017 which type of food or drink brought the most money into the UK from exports?

   a) fruit and veg *b) meat* *c) beverages*

3) Which country exports the most chocolate in the world?

   a) Germany *b) USA* *c) Belgium*

4) Turmeric is used in mustard to give it a yellowy colour:

   True or False?

5) Which of these isn't a fruit: apple, orange, tomato, rhubarb?
6) If you've cut vegetables 'julienne', what will they look like?
7) Which country was first to make and sell Hawaiian (ham and pineapple) pizzas?
8) What is 'cannelloni'?
9) Which country is the world's biggest olive producer, based on tons produced per year?

Therapy Targets

Answers for Activity 6 – Food quiz

1) The film title ends with …. **Meatballs**.

2) According to the Office for National Statistics, in 2017 which type of food or drink brought the most money into the UK from exports?

   a) Fruit and veg b) Meat **c) Beverages (whisky from Scotland)**

3) Which country exports the most chocolate in the world?

   a) Germany b) USA c) Belgium

   a) Germany (while the USA is said to produce the most chocolate, Germany exports more)

4) Turmeric is used in mustard to give it the yellowy colour:

   True or False?

5) Which of these isn't a fruit: apple, orange, tomato, **rhubarb**?

6) If you've cut vegetables 'julienne', what will they look like? **Thin strips**

7) Which country was first to make and sell Hawaiian (ham and pineapple) pizzas? **America – 'invented' by a Greek chef!**

8) What is 'cannelloni'? **Pasta tubes**

9) Which country is the world's biggest olive producer, based on tons produced per year? **Spain**

Therapy Targets

Activity 7(a): Synonyms (words provided)

Instructions: Look at the word on the left in **bold**. Underline the word in the same row that could be used to replace it.

drinks	beverages	dinner
food	fire	nourishment
bread	loaf	cake
sausages	bangers	bacon
cake	casserole	muffin
flan	quiche	fish
pasty	pizza	patty
wine	glass	vino
beer	ale	cider
curry	sweet and sour	Balti
sandwich	sarnie	egg

Do you have alternative words for the words on the left?

Therapy Targets

Activity 7(b): Synonyms

Instructions: Can you think of another word that means the same as each word below?

Drinks

Food

Bread

Sausages

Cake

Flan

Pasty

Wine

Beer

Curry

Sandwich

Chips

Can you think of any other food and drink synonyms?

Therapy Targets

Activity 8: Favourite food and drink

Instructions: Thinking about your favourite meal, answer the questions below.

- ❑ What do you like about it?
- ❑ Can you make it?
- ❑ How often do you eat it?
- ❑ What is your least favourite meal?

Now repeat for your favourite drink.

Therapy Targets

Activity: Words of increasing length

Instructions: Read across each row. Say the words. Use the words in the third column to make a longer sentence.

The blank boxes at the bottom can be used for your own word sequences.

One syllable	Two syllables	Multisyllabic	Now say a complete sentence using the multisyllabic word or phrase
Cook	Cooking	Cooking class	
Chop	Chopping	Chopping board	
Stir	Stirring	Stirring soup	
Grate	Grated	Grated cheese	
Chop	Chopsticks	Use chopsticks	
Drink	Drinking	Drinking tea	

Therapy Targets

CHAPTER 14

THEME: ENTERTAINMENT

CONTENTS				
ACTIVITY & PAGE NUMBER	**ACTIVITY**	**CLIENT GROUP**	**LEVEL**	**COMMENTS & SUGGESTIONS**
1 Page 184	Finding smaller words from a longer word	Language (especially word recall and spelling), group	L2–L3	
2 Page 185	Alphabetical word order – miscellaneous topics	Language (especially word recall and spelling), group	L2–L3	
3 Page 186	Word association – various topics	Language	L1–L2	
4 Page 187	ACROSTIC – film and theatre	Language, group	L3	
5(a) Page 188	Sentence completion (spoken)	All	L1	
5(b) Page 189	Sentence completion (written)	Language (written)	L1–L2	
5(c) Page 190	Sentence completion (spoken or written)	All	L2–L3	There might be more than one correct response.
6 Page 191	Theatre boardgame	All	L1	Make this a L3 activity – ask the person to make sentences from the words.
7 Page 192	Card game – various topics	All	L2–L3	
8 Page 193	Comparisons	All	L3	L2 people might manage this exercise with support. Use pictures/words to make this a L1 exercise.
9 Pages 194–195	Short story – a day out	All	L2–L3	

DOI: 10.4324/9781003177852-14

Activity 1: Finding smaller words from a longer word

Instructions: How many little words can you make from the word entertainment? The 'new' words do not have to be related to entertainment.

E N T E R T A I N M E N T

Therapy Targets

Activity 2: Alphabetical word order

Instructions: Put the words below into alphabetical order.

Theatre

Poetry

Ballet

Cinema

Films

Concert

Comedy

Bowling

Art gallery

Dance

Opera

Television

Games

Fireworks

Museum

Therapy Targets

Activity 3: Word association

Instructions: Match the words in the box below with the places in the list. You can use the words in the box wherever they apply.

play	music	comedy	bar	bowling
coffee	meal	film	drink	art

Art gallery

Television

Restaurant

Bar

Club

Theatre

Café

Bowling alley

Cinema

Concert hall

Therapy Targets

Activity 4: ACROSTIC

Instructions: Use each letter in the word to find new, related words or a phrase. Each new word or phrase begins with each letter of the given word.

Example: **FILM**

F – FICTION

I – IMAGINATION

L – LOVE

M – MOVIE

THEATRE

T –

H –

E –

A –

T –

R –

E –

Therapy Targets

Activity 5(a): Sentence completion (spoken)

Instructions: The therapist reads these sentences aloud to be completed by the client.

Ten pin _______________ (bowling)

Break a _______________ (leg)

MacDonald's meal _____________ (deal)

Roll the _______________ (dice)

These are the best seats in the ____________ (house)

Shuffle the _____________ (cards)

The comedian was very ______________ (funny)

The performance starts in 10 _____________ (minutes)

It's the opening _______________ (night)

Get out the red _______________ (carpet)

These coins are ancient _____________ (relics)

What's on the TV ______________ (tonight)

That painting is a master ______________ (piece)

Two for the price of _______________ (one)

Therapy Targets

Activity 5(b): Sentence completion (written)

Instructions: Read these sentences. Write out the word to complete the sentence.

Ten pin ___________

Break a ___________

MacDonald's meal ___________

Roll the ____________

These are the best seats in the ____________

Shuffle the __________

The comedian was very __________

The performance starts in 10 __________

It's the opening __________

Get out the red ___________

These coins are ancient ___________

What's on the TV ___________

That painting is a master __________

Two for the price of ____________

Therapy Targets

Activity 5(c): Sentence completion (spoken or written)

Instructions: Read these sentences. Complete each sentence. Write out or speak your answer.

I fancy a beer, let's go to the __________

What's on at the __________

Let's get tickets for ___________

It's raining, let's take the kids __________

I can't be bothered to cook, let's __________

Would you like to meet up for a ___________

I've reserved seats for ___________

There's a new exhibition, let's go to the ___________

Do you want to try the new ____________

On holiday, we could visit the ____________

It's two-for-one at the ____________

Therapy Targets

Activity 6: Theatre-themed board game

Instructions: Find a counter for each person, roll the dice and make your way around the board. Say the word written in the square you land on. Move to the box above when you land on a rising star actor; move to the box below when you land on a falling star.

36 FINALE	37	38 APPLAUSE	39	40 ENCORE	THE END
35	34	33 ROW	32	31 SCRIPT	30
24 ICE-CREAM	25	26 REHEARSAL	27 AUDIENCE	28	29 BALLET
23	22 DRINKS	21 BAR	20 INTERVAL	19 AISLE	18 USHER
12	13	14	15 LIGHTING	16	17
11 ACTOR	10 OPERA		9 CURTAINS	8	7 FINAL CALL
1 START	2 TICKET	3 CLOAKROOM	4	5 PERFORMANCE	6 SEAT

Therapy Targets

Activity 7: Card game

Instructions: Cut out the cards. Place the number cards face up in a column. Place the questions face down in a pile next to each corresponding number.

The client rolls a dice and picks up a question card matching the number they have rolled. E.g. roll a 6, pick up a music question card.

1 Theatre	Name the part of the stage actors stand on	What are the people who watch a play called?	When the play is about to begin, what opens in front of the stage?	To wish actors good luck on the first night of a play, you might say ______________
2 Bowling	What is the term used when somebody knocks over all the skittles?	What is a strike?	How many holes in a bowling ball?	In bowling, the balls are rolled down the bowling ______________
3 Eating Out	Name the place where you go for a meal	Name a place you go for a coffee	When choosing a meal, you look at the _________	The person who serves you is called a ____________
4 Art Gallery	Name a famous artist	A person who makes models from metal, wood and ice is called a ____	Name a famous art gallery	A picture produced from oils onto canvas is called an oil _________
5 Cinema	What might you eat whilst watching a film?	When a film is shown for the first time, it is called the ____	On the opening night of a film, the actors walk down the ____	A film where a couple fall in love is called a ________
6 Music	Which radio station plays classical music?	Name a station that plays pop music	Name a music genre	Name a musical instrument

Therapy Targets

Activity 8: Comparisons

Instructions: Describe the similarities and differences between the terms below.

Theatre – Cinema

Café – Restaurant

Audience – Actor

Museum – Art gallery

Parade – Demonstration

Ballet – Opera

Actor – Comedian

Therapy Targets

Activity 9(a): Short story – a day out

Instructions: See the following page for suggestions on how to use the story.

The Green family were on holiday. It was a grey day, and it would be too cold to go to the beach. They decided to visit the local sites of interest instead. Over breakfast, they planned their day. Jo was keen to see the old harbour and look at some of the yachts and ships moored up by the old lighthouse. He'd glimpsed a large, red ship and was fascinated by its size. The rest of the family agreed to go to the harbour, provided they could go to the art gallery first.

Once mum had made her flask of strong, black coffee, they set off. The blue hire car trundled its way through the ancient, cobbled streets until they reached the little gallery tucked away in a quaint old courtyard.

Inside the art gallery, the family were not disappointed. There were old and modern masterpieces. Dad decided that the piece entitled 'white blank space' was not to his taste. He declared he was hungry, so the family made their way to the little café in the courtyard. Coffees and irresistible cakes were ordered.

When they had finished their drinks and cakes, they headed to the harbour, just as the red ship sailed away! But Jo was not to be disappointed; there were plenty of other vessels to look at, including a gleaming silver, state of the art motor cruiser.

Activity 9(b): Short story – suggestions for use

Instructions: Use the short story in Activity 9(a).

1) Read the story aloud for speech, voice or fluency practice.
2) As a language activity, ask the person to underline different word categories, e.g. colours, adjectives, verbs or nouns.
3) Read the passage to the person, then ask them questions about it.
4) Provide the short story along with a series of written questions.
5) Ask the person to write about a day out they have enjoyed.

Therapy Targets

Activity: Words of increasing length

Instructions: Read across each row. Say the words. Use the words in the third column to make a longer sentence.

One syllable	Two syllables	Multisyllabic	Now say a complete sentence using the multisyllabic word or phrase
Pub	Public	Public house	
Dance	Dancing	Go dancing	
Bowl	Bowling	Bowling alley	
Con	Concert	Concert tickets	
Act	Actor	Great actor	
Men	Menu	See the menu	

The blank boxes at the bottom can be used for your own word sequences.

Therapy Targets

CHAPTER 15

THEME: FOOTBALL

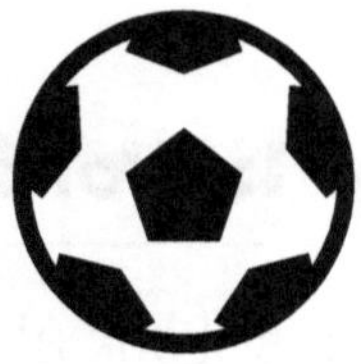

CONTENTS				
ACTIVITY & PAGE NUMBER	**ACTIVITY**	**CLIENT GROUP**	**LEVEL**	**COMMENTS**
1 Pages 198–199	Word search	Language	L1	
2 Pages 200–201	Word search – team members	Language	L2–L3	
3 Page 202	Describe team roles	All	L2–L3	
4(a) Page 203	Types of football shots	Language	L1	Make this a L3 activity – ask the client to describe what the shots mean.
4(b) Page 204	Types of football shots – definitions	Language	L3	
5 Page 205	Ideas-web: football	Language, speech	L2–L3	
6 Page 206	Football equipment – alphabetical ordering	Language	L2	
7 Page 207	Football equipment – definitions	All	L2–L3	
8 Pages 208–209	Football equipment – pairs game	All	L1–L2	
9 Page 210	Discussion topics	All	L2–L3	

DOI: 10.4324/9781003177852-15

Activity 1: Word search – words provided

Instructions: Look at the words below. Can you find them in the letter grid on the next page?

ball

score

team

goal

player

Can you find any other, non-football words?

Therapy Targets

Activity 1(b): Word search – no words provided

Instructions: How many football words can you find in the letter grid?

T	S	C	O	R	E	T	R
R	E	D	N	S	A	E	U
Q	E	X	N	G	C	A	M
Y	A	Y	L	O	Z	M	B
H	O	P	A	A	T	D	K
L	L	A	B	L	T	I	N
S	B	U	K	I	P	E	N

Therapy Targets

Activity 2: Word search – team members

Instructions: Look at the words below. Can you find team roles in the letter grid on the next page?

goalkeeper

referee

manager

linesman

midfielder

attacker

substitute

fan

defender

coach

captain

There are 5 other football related words in the word search. Can you find them?

Therapy Targets

Activity 2: Word search – team members

G	H	Z	B	C	A	P	T	A	I	N	E	H	C	K	L
G	R	B	H	D	B	V	H	S	N	A	A	L	W	S	I
J	O	G	D	I	A	R	L	M	R	C	N	F	U	O	A
P	K	A	T	E	L	T	R	E	F	E	R	E	E	H	T
C	S	M	L	U	L	L	A	O	G	T	W	F	H	N	T
R	H	J	D	K	A	F	G	N	Y	J	V	C	F	G	A
R	H	J	D	E	E	D	F	V	G	H	A	J	L	F	C
E	G	H	J	N	K	E	Y	S	U	O	I	O	I	P	K
D	B	S	D	B	G	U	P	K	C	S	D	F	N	Q	E
L	S	P	I	T	C	H	G	E	E	O	M	R	E	K	R
E	U	N	W	J	T	H	A	X	R	K	R	D	S	F	N
I	E	N	S	U	B	S	T	I	T	U	T	E	M	Z	V
F	D	P	R	T	U	C	S	K	D	Y	F	T	A	U	H
D	X	R	E	G	A	N	A	M	X	H	K	D	N	M	E
I	D	W	V	J	A	A	D	H	M	A	T	C	H	R	J
M	Q	A	D	D	E	F	E	N	D	E	R	R	L	C	U

Therapy Targets

Activity 3: Describe team roles

Instructions: Describe the role of each member of the team.

goalkeeper

referee

manager

linesman

midfielder

attacker

substitute

fan

defender

coach

captain

Therapy Targets

Activity 4(a): Types of football shots

Instructions: Identify which of the moves below are football shots.

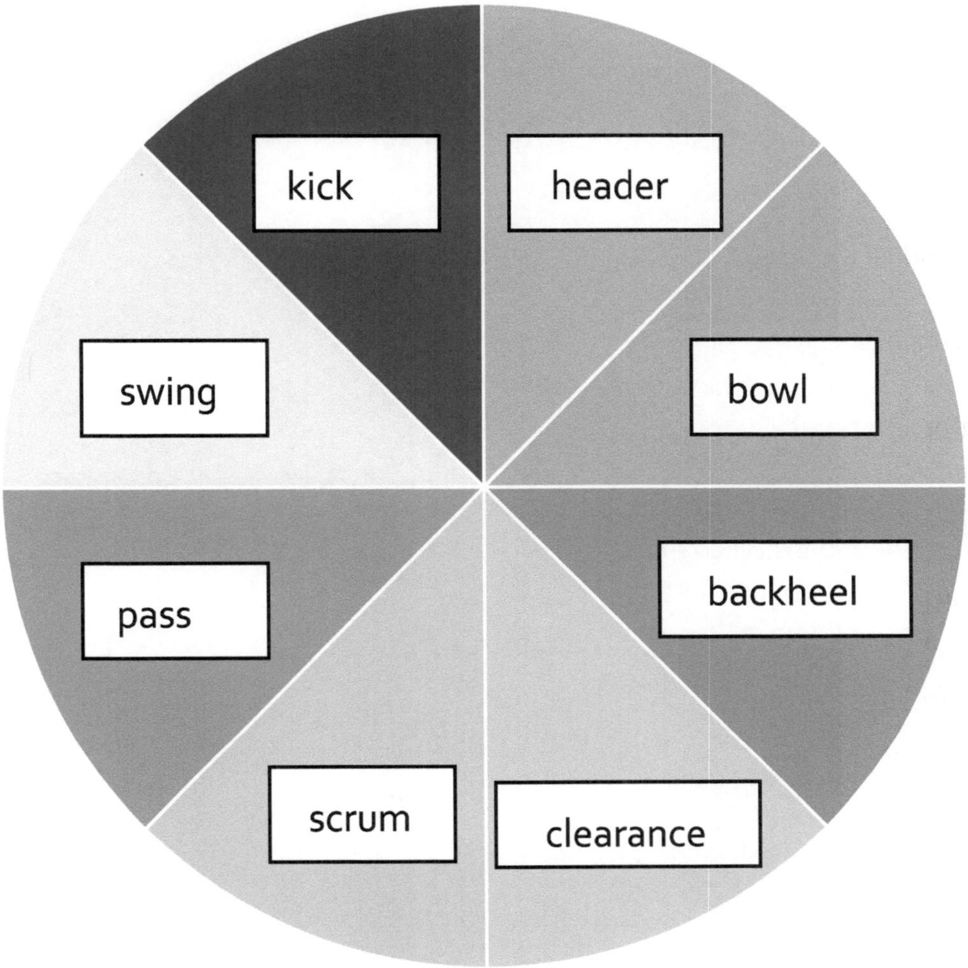

Can you name four more football shots?

Therapy Targets

Activity 4(b): Types of football shots (definitions)

Instructions: Define these football shots.

A pass

A volley

A kick

A backheel

A clearance

A header

A cross

A penalty

A throw-in

A shoot

Therapy Targets

Activity 5: Ideas-web: football

Instructions: Answer the questions below.

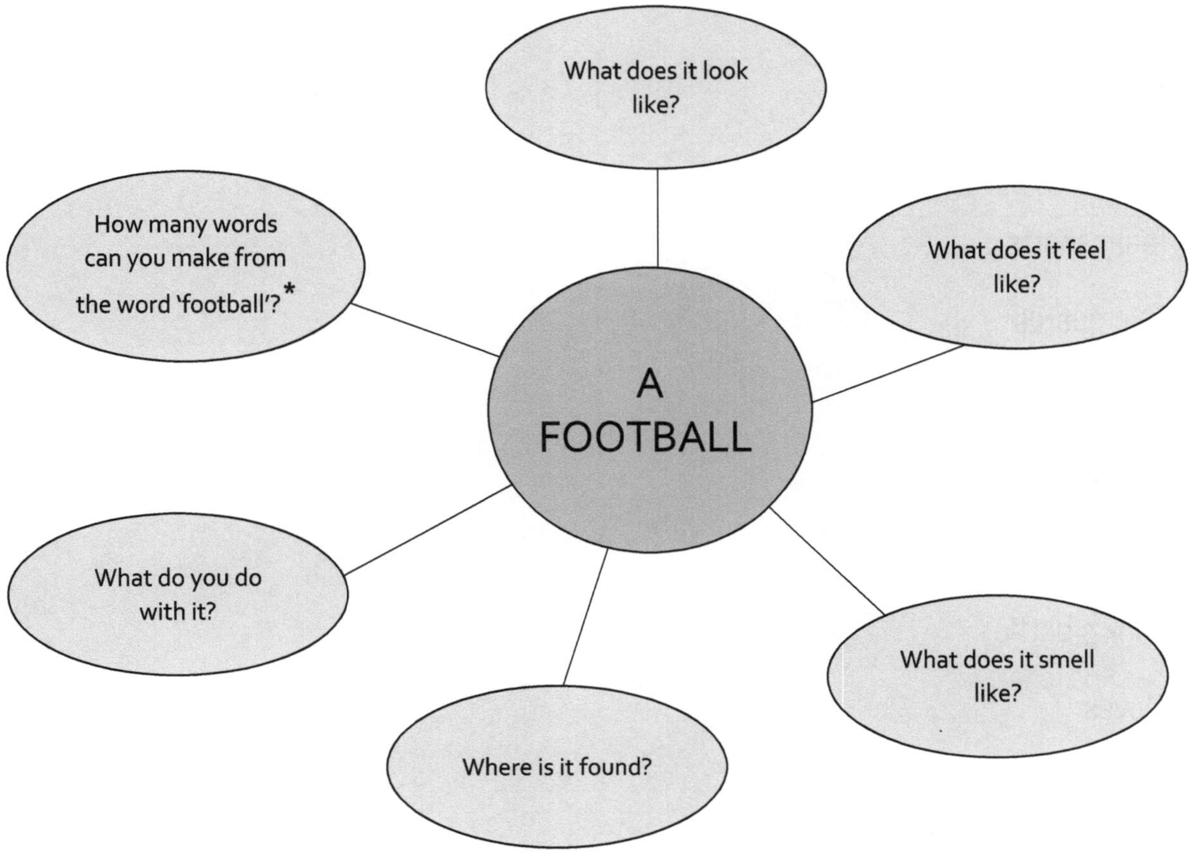

Repeat the exercise above using these words:

Football pitch

Football shirt

** (the words do not have to be football related)*

Therapy Targets

Activity 6: Football equipment – alphabetical ordering

Instructions: Put these words into alphabetical order.

Grip socks

Studs

Team shirt

Team shorts

Shin guards

Deodorant

Towel

Shoes

Drink's bottle

Gloves

Hat

Jacket

Flip-flops

Boot freshener

Sock tape

Ankle guards

Football

Kit bag

Therapy Targets

Activity 7: Football equipment – definitions

Instructions: What is each item of football equipment used for?

Grip socks

Studs

Team shirt

Team shorts

Shin guards

Deodorant

Towel

Shoes

Drink's bottle

Gloves

Hat

Jacket

Flip-flops

Boot freshener

Sock tape

Ankle guards

Football

Kit bag

Therapy Targets

Activity 8: Football equipment

Instructions: See activity ideas on the following page.

Grip socks	Studs	Team shirt
Team shorts	Shin guards	Deodorant
Towel	Shoes	Drink's bottle
Gloves	Hat	Jacket
Flip-flops	Boot freshener	Sock tape
Ankle guards	Football	Kit bag

Therapy Targets

Activity 8: Football equipment – pairs game

Instructions: There are several ways to use the 'cards' on the previous page.

Print off two copies of the word grid and cut the squares into individual 'cards'.

i) Pairs game
Place the word pairs face-down on a table. Mix the cards up. Take it in turns to turn over two cards until you find a pair.

ii) Pairs game with speech
Play as above and say the word each time it is turned over.

iii) Dice game

- ❑ Number the backs of the cards, 1 to 6. Repeat this twice more. You will now have 3 sets of cards, each labelled 1–6. Arrange the cards into groups according to number so you have a pile of cards marked as 1 another as 2 and so on.
- ❑ Turn the cards over so you can only see the numbers.
- ❑ Take it in turns to roll a dice and select a card matching the number you have rolled.
- ❑ Depending on the therapy target and level for the person, ask them to:
  - a) say the word
  - b) put the word into a sentence
  - c) define it
- ❑ Put the used card aside.

Therapy Targets

Activity 9: Discussion topics

Instructions: Use the discussion ideas below according to the therapy target (e.g. using full sentences, using loud voice etc).

Discussion ideas:

Which football team do you support?

Why do you support them?

How long have you supported them?

Where are they based?

Do they have a mascot?

Who are their most feared opponents?

Where are they in the league table currently?

What is the highest they have climbed in the leagues?

What are their colours this season?

Therapy Targets

Activity: Words of increasing length

Instructions: Read across each row. Say the words. Use the words in the third column to make a longer sentence.

The blank boxes at the bottom can be used for your own word sequences.

One syllable	Two syllables	Multisyllabic	Now say a complete sentence using the multisyllabic word or phrase
Foot	Football	Football club	
Kick	Kicking	Kicking the ball	
Head	Header	Good header	
Score	Scoring	Scoring a goal	
Play	Player	Top player	
Cap	Captain	New captain	

Therapy Targets

CHAPTER 16

THEME: THE GREAT OUTDOORS

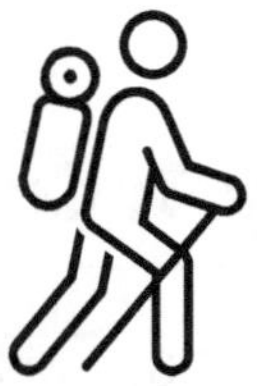

CONTENTS

ACTIVITY & PAGE NUMBER	ACTIVITY	CLIENT GROUP	LEVEL	COMMENTS & SUGGESTIONS
1 Page 214	Camping – memory and word recall	All	L2–L3	Excellent group exercise. L1 clients could select written words or pictures.
2(a) Page 215	In my rucksack – word recall		L1	
2(b) Page 216	In my rucksack – word recall		L1	
2(c) Page 217	In my rucksack – word recall		L2 - L3	
3 Page 218	Story completion	All	L3	
4 Page 219	Categories of outdoor activities	Language, group	L2 – L3	
5 Page 220	Discussion – your favourite activity or sport	All	L2–L3	L2 people might need supported communication to participate.
6 Page 221	Describing outdoor activities	All	L2–L3	
7 Page 222	Comparisons	All	L3	
8 Page 223	Missing words	Language, speech, voice, fluency	L2	
9(a) Page 224	Draw or mime the action	Language	L1	
9(b) Page 225	Draw or mime the object	Language	L1	
10 Page 226	What colour am I?	Language, speech	L1–L2	L1 people might need colour cards to support them.

DOI: 10.4324/9781003177852-16

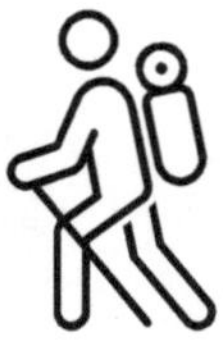

Activity 1: Camping – memory and word recall game

Instructions: Take it in turns to say, 'I went camping and forgot to take …'. Try to remember the previous peoples' items.

TIP: Use gestures to help remind each other which items have been named so far.

'I went camping and forgot to take … …' .

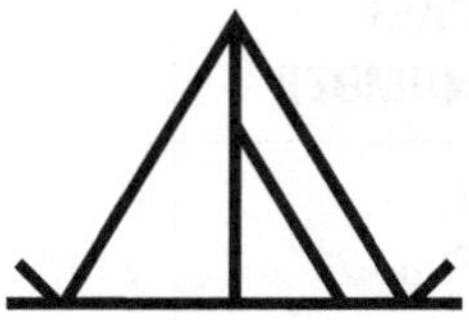

Therapy Targets

Activity 2(a): In my rucksack – word recall

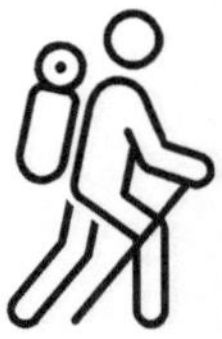

Instructions: Name or write the items you would put into your rucksack for a long walk or a day trip. Use the pictures to help you.

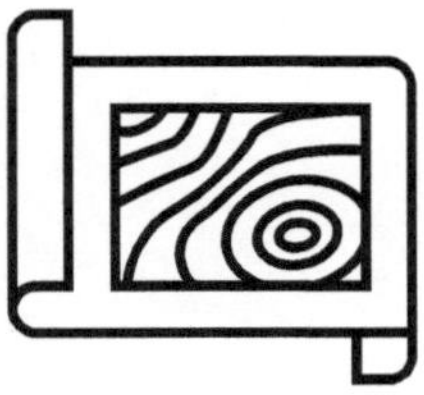

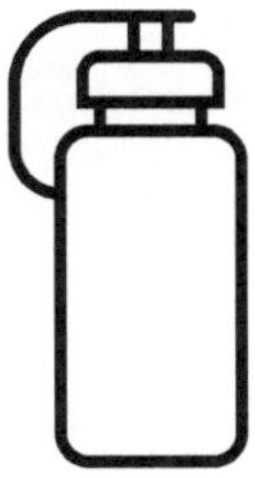

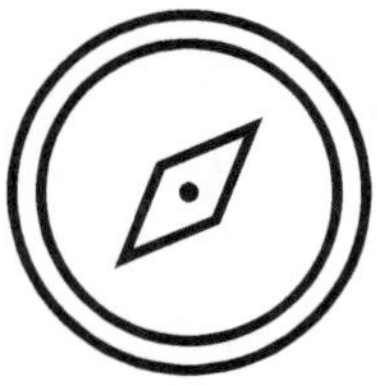

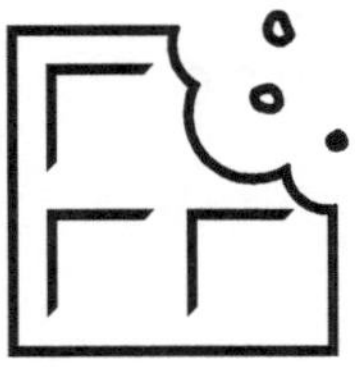

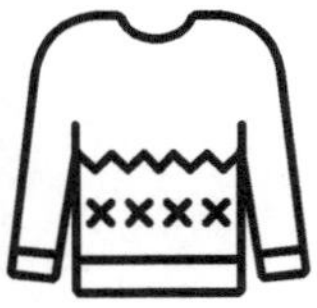

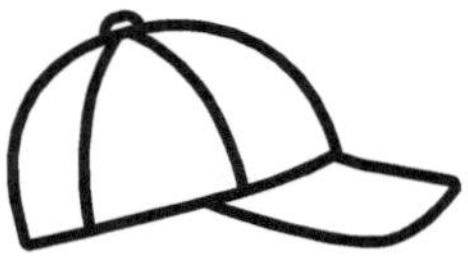

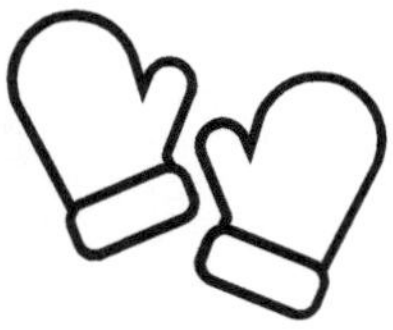

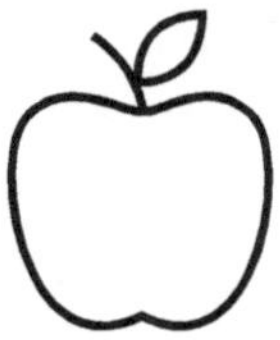

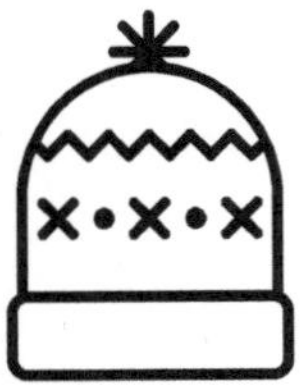

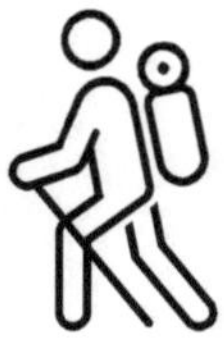

Activity 2(b): In my rucksack – word recall

Instructions: Unscramble the letters to name the items you might put into your rucksack for a long walk or a day trip.

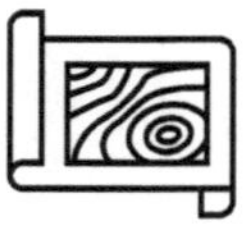 p a m

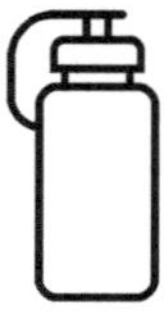 n i k d r

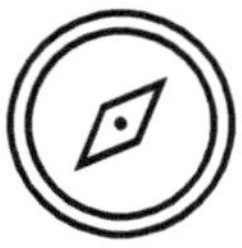 s a s m p c o

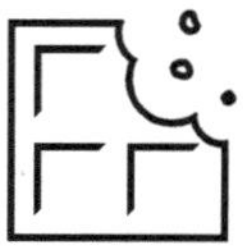 h c o c l a e t o

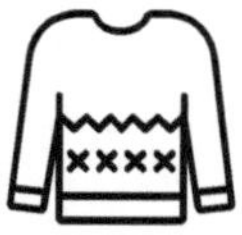 m u p r e j

 d e r a b

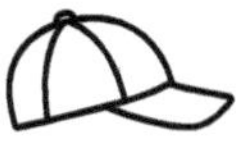 a p c

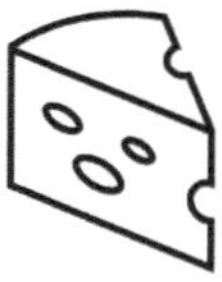 h e s e h c

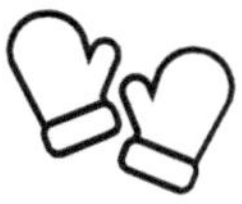 t i m t e s n

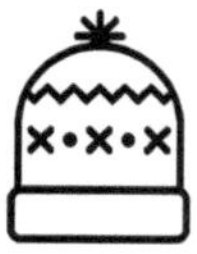 t a h

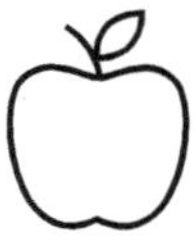 p p e l a

Therapy Targets

Activity 2(c): In my rucksack – word recall

Instructions: Say or write out a list of items you would put into your rucksack for a long walk or a day trip.

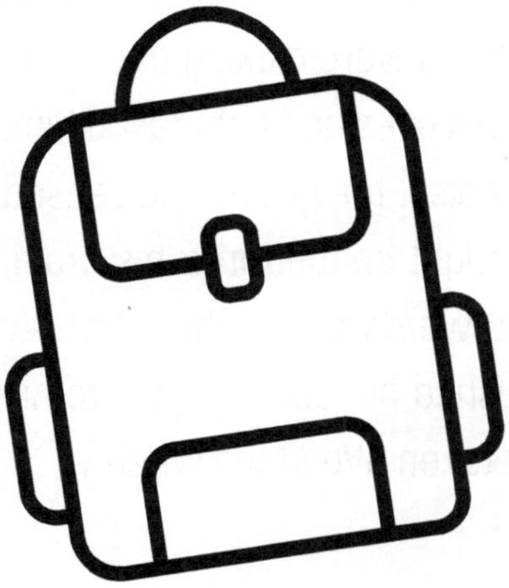

Therapy Targets

Activity 3: Story completion

Instructions: Read the story below and think of a suitable ending.

It was a hot and heavy day, and he had been walking for over two hours. He sat down on a moss-covered log to have a drink. As he sat in the woodland clearing, he could smell the rotting leaves underfoot and hear the rustling of hidden creatures moving in the nearby bushes. He strained his eyes to see which creatures were making the noise. He listened carefully to locate the source of the noise, but his eyes and ears failed him. The harder he tried to see and hear what was making the noise, the greater he sensed that something was about to change forever. As this thought seeped into his brain, he became aware of a growing urge to follow the path towards the bushes that lay temptingly ahead of him. He rose purposefully, quickly pushed his belongings into his old rucksack and set off towards the bushes. He had only taken five steps when … .

Therapy Targets

Activity 4: Categories of outdoor activities

Instructions: Match the activity to the category.

sailing	BASE-jumping	skiing	abseiling
mountain biking	via ferratas	kayaking	sledging
snowboarding	running	climbing	coasteering
ice climbing	horse riding	orienteering	surfing

Water Sports	Land Sports
Winter Sports	**Extreme Sports**

Therapy Targets

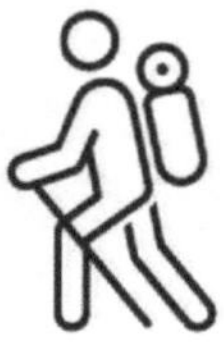

Activity 5: Discussion – your favourite outdoor activity or sport

Instructions: Describe your favourite outdoor activity.

TIP: Some points to consider are given below.

- ❑ Why you like it.
- ❑ Is it a solo sport or a team activity?
- ❑ Can you do it near to where you live, or do you have to travel?
- ❑ How often do you manage to do your sport?
- ❑ What special equipment do you need to do your sport?

Therapy Targets

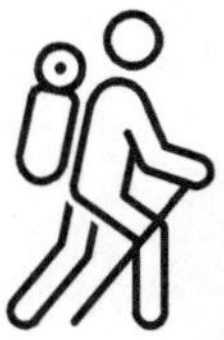

Activity 6: Describing outdoor activities

Instructions: Describe these outdoor activities. i.e. What are they?

Coasteering

Snowboarding

Bird-watching

Climbing

Mountain biking

Kayaking

Sledging

Horse riding

Walking

Scrambling

Therapy Targets

Activity 7: Comparisons

Instructions: Describe the similarities and differences between the terms below.

Climbing – Scrambling

Kayaking – Canoeing

Bird-watching – Shooting

Sledging – Skiing

Sailing – Windsurfing

Bodyboarding – SUP boarding

Therapy Targets

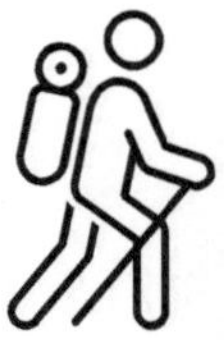

Activity 8: Missing words

Instructions: Using the words from the box, complete the passage below.

coast	pulling	sun	hard	bay	kayaks
seals	stronger	food	morning	out	busy

We decided to take the ________ into the sea and paddle around the __________. We set off early in the __________ before the beach became too _______. As the tide was going out, paddling was _______ work and after an hour we stopped to have a drink and some __________.

As we set off again, we spotted some ______ swimming in the water. We could see their heads bobbing about as they watched us. We moved further around the head-land and the swell became _______. We could also feel the current __________ us away from the shoreline. We carried on paddling until we could see the ______ where we were getting __________. The beach seemed a long time coming, but finally we were sat on the sand, enjoying the warmth of the _______. What a great paddle!

Therapy Targets

Activity 9(a): Draw or mime the action

Instructions: Cut out the word cards below and place them face down on the table.

Take it in turns to pick up a card without showing each other.

Draw or mime the action for the other person to guess.

Reading a map	Kayaking
Climbing	Putting up a tent
Horse riding	Running
Orienteering	Bird-watching
Lighting a fire	Sleeping in a cold tent

Therapy Targets

Activity 9(b): Draw or mime the object

Instructions: Cut out the word cards below and place them face down on the table.

Take it in turns to pick up a card without showing each other.

Draw or mime the object for the other person to guess.

Kayak	Rucksack
Tent	Map
Flask	Surfboard
Bird	Hat
Binoculars	River

Therapy Targets

Activity 10: What colour am I?

Instructions: Write or say what colour the following items are.

Snow

Sun

Sky

Clouds

Sea

Grass

Squirrel

Mud

Sheep

Heather

Daffodils

Therapy Targets

Activity: Words of increasing length

Instructions: Read across each row. Say the words. Use the words in the third column to make a longer sentence.

The blank boxes at the bottom can be used for your own word sequences.

One syllable	Two syllables	Multisyllabic	Now say a complete sentence using the multisyllabic word or phrase
Camp	Camping	Camping holiday	
Climb	Climbing	Climbing shoes	
Bike	Biking	Mountain biking	
Pick	Picnic	Have a picnic	
Out	Outdoors	Let's go outdoors	
Ram	Rambling	He goes rambling	

Therapy Targets

CHAPTER 17

THEME: RACQUETS, BATS AND BALLS

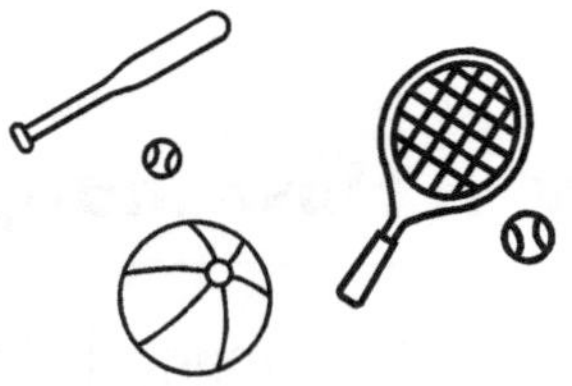

CONTENTS				
ACTIVITY & PAGE NUMBER	ACTIVITY	CLIENT GROUP	LEVEL	COMMENTS & SUGGESTIONS
1 Page 230	How many smaller words in a longer word?	All	L2–L3	
2 Page 231	Sorting words into categories	Language	L1–L2	
3 Page 232	Team roles	All	L3	
4(a) Page 233	Ideas-web: racquet	All	L2–L3	
4(b) Page 234	Ideas-web: bat	All	L2–L3	
5 Page 235	A–Z of racquets, bats and balls	All Especially good as a group/quiz	L2–L3	In a group, split the group into two teams – who can find the most words per letter?
6 Page 236	Beat the batsman game	Language – spelling; group	L2–L3	Good for two or more clients working together.
7 Page 237	Word table tennis	All	L1–L3	
8 Page 238	Phrase completion	All	L1	
9 Pages 239–240	Question grid	All	L1–L2	Good group game.
10 Page 241	Word identification	Language	L1	Could be read by the person, or spoken aloud for the person to write or speak their answer.

DOI: 10.4324/9781003177852-17

Activity 1: How many smaller words in a longer word?

Instructions: How many little words can you find in the word BADMINTON?

B A D M I N T O N

Can you put each of those words into different sentences?

How many of those words can you put into one sentence?

Therapy Targets

Activity 2: Sorting words into categories

Instructions: Decide whether each of the sports below is a 'net' game or a 'bat' game.

tennis rounders netball cricket

table tennis badminton basketball

volleyball baseball hockey

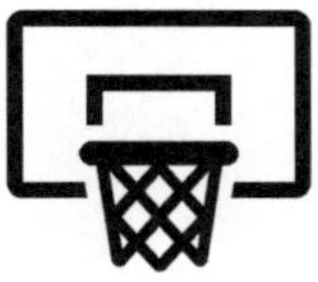

net game

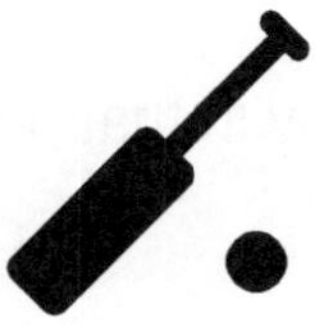

bat game

Therapy Targets

Activity 3: Team roles

Instructions: Name the different team positions in a sport of your choice and explain their roles.

If you play (or played) in a team, what position do (did) you play?

Do you like that position?

Why do (did) you play in that position?

Therapy Targets

Activity 4(a): Ideas-web – racquet

Instructions: Answer the questions in the balls, about a racquet.

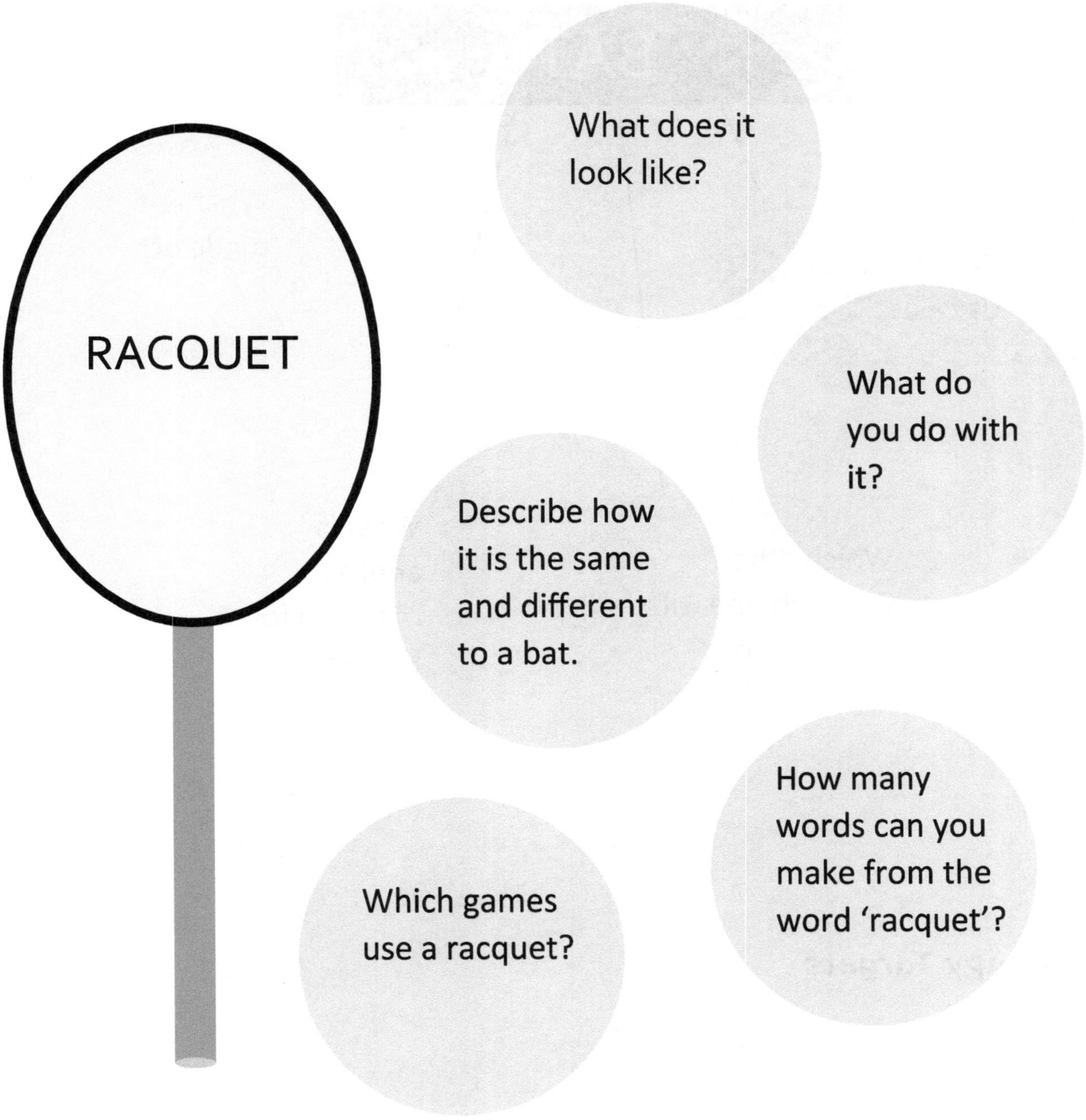

Therapy Targets

Activity 4(b): Ideas-web – bat

Instructions: Answer the questions below, about a bat.

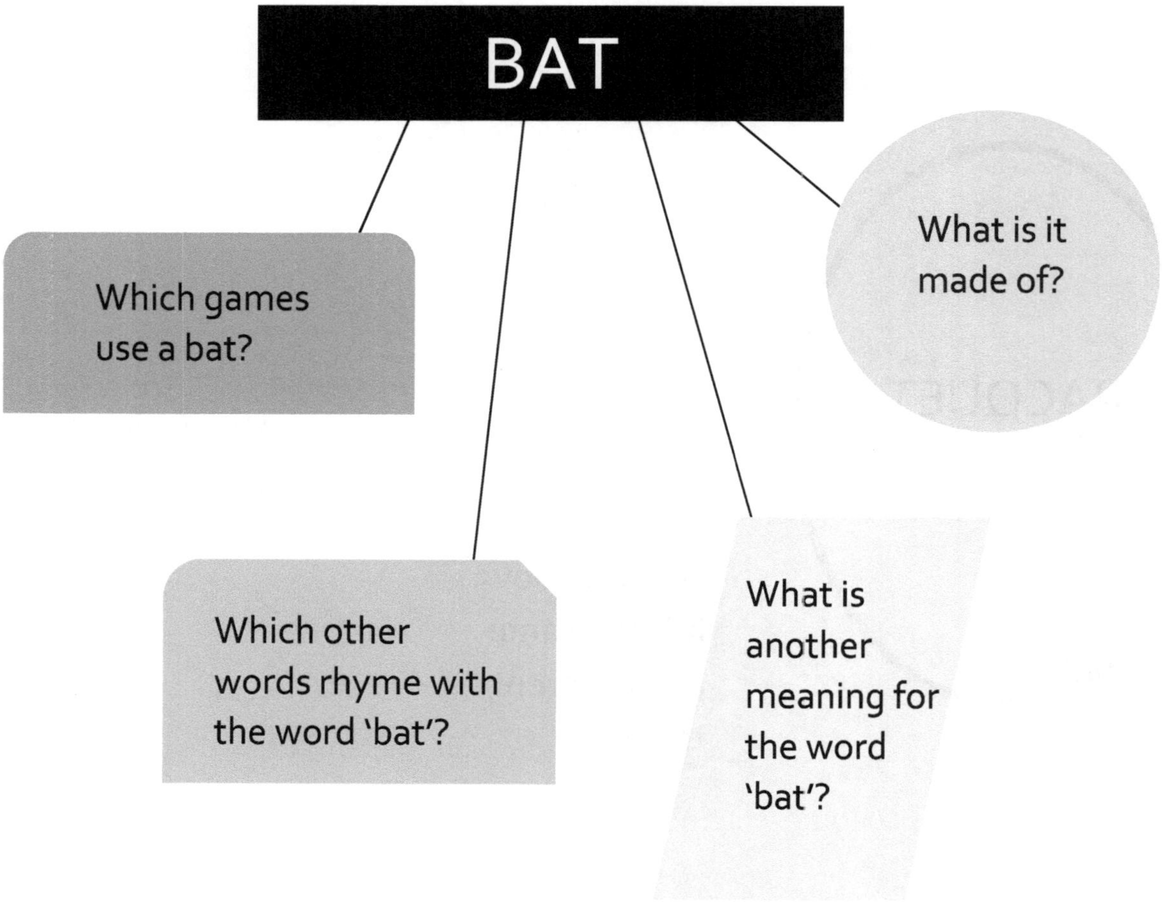

Therapy Targets

Activity 5: A–Z of racquets, bats and balls

Instructions: Go through the alphabet and name something related to racquets, bats and balls for each letter.

Creative answers and famous player names are allowed!

A		N	
B		O	
C		P	
D		Q	
E		R	
F		S	
G		T	
H		U	
I		V	
J		W	
K		X	
L		Y	
M		Z	

Therapy Targets

Activity 6: Beat the batsman

Instructions: Think of a word related to a sport, e.g. 'deuce' and follow the steps below.

- ❑ Don't tell the other person your word.
- ❑ Can they guess your word?
- ❑ Can the word be guessed before you have completed drawing the batsman (like the one below)?
- ❑ You need to draw:
  - A head • two arms • a body • two legs • a bat • the bat handle • the bat body
  - three balls
- ❑ It might help to draw a line for each letter in your word. E.g. bat would have three lines:

  __ __ __
- ❑ Cross out each letter as it is said.

A B C D E F G H I J K L M N O P Q R S T U V W X Y Z

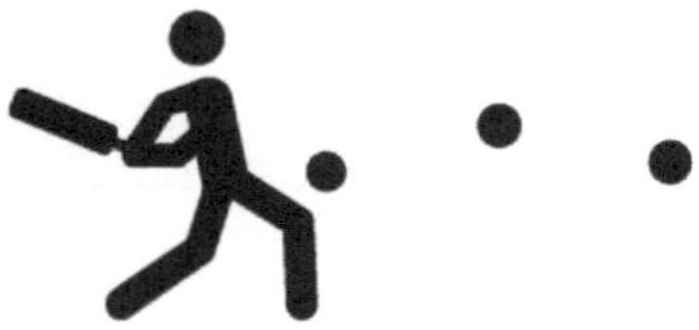

Therapy Targets

Activity 7: Word table tennis

Instructions: The first person thinks of a word and says it out loud. The next person says another word associated with the first word.

Bounce the ideas between the players, each time saying a word associated to the previous word.

Example:

> "Tennis – ball – round – circle – square – chocolate – brown – mud – slippery – falling – bruise – blue – sky".

You could start with one of the following words or think of your own.

Cricket

Weather

Volleyball

Therapy Targets

Activity 8: Phrase completion

Instructions: Complete the phrases below.

Bat and ___________ (ball)

All out for __________ (one)

Fifteen _____________ (love)

In the _____________ (net)

It's a sticky ___________ (wicket)

Game, set and ___________ (match)

That's bad! He got a red ____________ (card)

A drop ____________ (shot)

Therapy Targets

Activity 9: Question grid

Instructions: See the following page for instructions on how to use the question grid.

6	In which game do you have a 'home run'?	What is the colour of a tennis ball?	How many nets in a netball game?	'Love' is a score in baseball. True or false?	What rhymes with 'bat'?	Name a racquet game
5	Name a piece of cricket equipment	Miss a go!	Name a position in cricket.	Name a game that uses a bat.	Roll again!	Which game uses a ping-pong ball?
4	Name a place you might play volleyball.	What word rhymes with 'net'?	What rhymes with 'ball'?	The colour of a table tennis ball	Badminton is good to play outside in the wind. True or false?	Name a famous tennis player.
3	Ask another player a question.	Name a piece of tennis equipment?	Name a sport for 2 or 4 players	Name an item of cricket clothing	Which bat and ball game is popular in America?	Choose a question to answer
2	'Deuce' means 'draw'. True or false?	The colour of a cricket ball	Miss a go!	Name a game that uses a net	Name a sport which is for two teams	How many players in rounders?
1	Name a famous tennis court	Roll again!	In which sport do they play for the Ashes?	What is hit between players in badminton?	Which ball games require helmets?	Miss a go!
	1	2	3	4	5	6

Therapy Targets

Activity 9: Question grid – how to use

Instructions: Follow the steps below.

1) Roll a dice – note the number.

2) Roll the dice again – note the number.

3) Now use the numbers to find your place on the grid, e.g. a 3 then a 2 is marked by an 'x' in the box below.

3		x	
2			
1			
	1	2	3

4) Answer the question in that box.

   If playing with more than one person, award points:

   i) one point for each correct answer or,

   ii) the score could be the numbers on the dice added up. In the example above, a two and a three = five.

Therapy Targets

Activity 10: Word identification

Instructions: Underline the words that are (select one):

Action words ☐ Object names ☐ Colours ☐

bowling	bat	quickly	blue
yellow	ball	tackling	hot
windy	green	serve	defending
net	catching	red	out
white	slicing	behind	shuttlecock
batting	glove	gold	competitive
black	shooting	sixty	team

Therapy Targets

Activity: Words of increasing length

Instructions: Read across each row. Say the words. Use the words in the third column to make a longer sentence.

The blank boxes at the bottom can be used for your own word sequences.

One syllable	Two syllables	Multisyllabic	Now say a complete sentence using the multisyllabic word or phrase
Bat	Batting	Batting the ball	
Bowl	Bowler	Fast bowler	
Hit	Hitting	Hitting the ball	
Shut	Shuttle	Shuttlecock	
Base	Baseball	Baseball player	
Ten	Tennis	Tennis match	

Therapy Targets

THEME: ARTS & CRAFTS

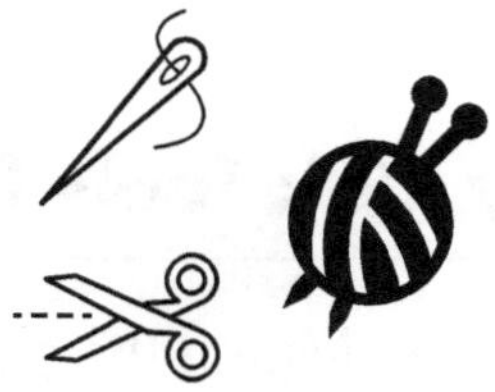

CONTENTS

DOI: 10.4324/9781003177852-18

Activity 1(a): Tools for crafts

Instructions: Match the craft with its tool.

Knitting	Parchment paper
Crocheting	Potter's wheel
Painting	Pencils
Cross stitch	Knitting needles
Pottery	Piping bag
Calligraphy	Crochet hook
Drawing	Bowl and wooden spoon
Cake decorating	Paint brush
Baking	Needle

Therapy Targets

Activity 1(b): Tools for crafts

Instructions: Which craft do you like? What tools do you need for your craft?

My favourite craft is______________________________

The tools for your craft:

1)

2)

3)

4)

5)

Therapy Targets

Activity 2: Painting

Instructions: List below the types of objects you could paint.

1)

2)

3)

4)

5)

What colour would you use for each item?

Therapy Targets

Activity 3: What are these made from?

Instructions: Name what these items are made from, i.e. what are their primary constituents, or what are they derived from? There might be more than one answer for each item.

Paper

Wool

Knitting needles

Sewing needles

Pencils

Thread

Icing

Paint

Fabric

Artificial flowers

Beads

Therapy Targets

Activity 4: The Knitting Corner

Instructions: Answer the questions below.

1) Describe how to knit a scarf.

2) Describe how to knit a jumper.

3) What ply wool do you prefer to knit with?

4) Do you knit following a pattern or can you knit without?

5) Name two knitting stitches.

Therapy Targets

Activity 5: The Painting Society

Instructions: Answer the questions below.

1) Which painting medium do you use?

2) What do you like to paint?

3) Who is your favourite artist?

4) When did you begin to paint?

5) Do you do any other arts or crafts?

6) The paint palette – name the colours of the rainbow.

Therapy Targets

Activity 6: Anagrams

Instructions: Unscramble the words to complete the sentences.

Thread the _____________ (d e l e n e)

Cut out the _____________ (n a t t r e p)

Spray over the stencil with ___________ (n p a i t)

Thread the beads onto the __________ (r w e i)

Pour the wax into the _____________ (m l u d o)

Melt the ____________ (x a w)

Bend the wire with the _____________ (l i p r s e)

Don't drop a ___________ (t i s h c t)

3-ply ___________ (l o w o)

Crochet ___________ (h k o o)

Crochet hooks used to be made from _________ (v r i o y)

She covered the chairs with new _________ (a r b i f c)

She threw a new pot out of ____________ (l y c a)

Therapy Targets

Activity 7: Colours of the palette

Instructions: Complete these phrases.

As white as __________

At the end of the ____________

Red sky at night, shepherd's __________

Red sky in the morning, shepherd's ___________

Once in a blue _______

Every cloud has a silver ____________

He was black and blue all ________

Green with __________

It's a red rag to a _______

Rose tinted __________

He's going to paint the town _______

She's a shrinking _______

A bolt from the ___________

Tickled __________

Therapy Targets

Activity 8: Crafts word search

Instructions: Find these words in the word search below:

card	glue	clay	needle	stamp	fabric
hook	scissors	beads	ribbon	scrapbook	

K	S	G	X	A	H	O	O	K
R	I	B	B	O	N	F	O	Q
P	M	A	T	S	M	O	C	N
Y	W	C	I	R	B	A	F	E
A	R	T	C	P	K	B	B	E
L	J	Z	A	G	L	U	E	D
C	N	R	R	M	D	L	A	L
I	C	E	D	U	H	E	D	E
S	C	I	S	S	O	R	S	D

Therapy Targets

Activity 9: Don't drop a stitch question game

Instructions: Roll a dice, then roll it again. Use both numbers to locate your question in the grid. Score a point for each question answered correctly.

6	What do you keep your knitting in?	Name a knitting stitch	What is the biggest item you have knitted?	How many strands of wool in 2-ply?	What is another name for wool?	What are wool slubs?
5	You dropped a stitch, lose 1 point	What animals give us wool?	How many smaller words can you make from 'knitted'	You are ahead of schedule, add a point	What is the 'gauge' or tension, in a knitting pattern?	You have lost your pattern, miss a go!
4	Say: 'Nina needed ninety green knitting needles'	What jumpers have a cable pattern?	Name a household item you could knit	What is the term for mending a hole in a sock?	Which is thicker, 2-ply or 3-ply?	Name a type of knitting needle
3	What does CO mean in a knitting pattern?	What's the name of the cover put on a teapot?	What is DK?	You dropped 2 stitches, lose 2 points	Name an item of clothing that can be knitted.	What else can you do with wool?
2	What is wool from a (certain type of) goat called?	You have lost your needles, miss a go!	What is a Fair Isle pattern?	What size needles would you use for knitting in DK?	What is the smallest item you have knitted?	How many strands of wool in 3-ply?
1	What does BO mean?	Name an item of clothing you would not knit!	Name a make of wool (company who produce it)	What is 'frogging'?	Name something you might knit for a baby	What might you sew on to the front of a cardigan so it can be 'done up'?
	1	2	3	4	5	6

Therapy Targets

Activity 9: Don't drop a stitch question game – answers

6	Bag, basket.	Purl		2	Yarn	Knobbly bits added to the wool to give it texture
5	You dropped a stitch, lose 1 point	Sheep Yaks Llamas Alpacas	kin, tin, ten, kit, net, den, kitted, dent, tent		The number of stitches & rows per inch	
4	Ask the person to say it quickly 5 times	Aran sweaters	Blanket, tea-cosy, cushion cover	Darning	3-ply	Single point, double point, circular
3	Cast On		Double Knit	You dropped 2 stitches, lose 2 points	Jumper, cardigan, scarf, hat	Crochet felting finger knitting
2	Cashmere		A row knitted in 2 different colours	4.5 – 5.5		3
1	Bind Off	Trousers, shirt, pants		To unravel your knitting	Cardigan, booties, bonnet	Buttons
	1	2	3	4	5	6

Activity: Words of increasing length

Instructions: Read across each row. Say the words. Use the words in the third column to make a longer sentence.

The blank boxes at the bottom can be used for your own word sequences.

One syllable	Two syllables	Multisyllabic	Now say a complete sentence using the multisyllabic word or phrase
Knit	Knitting	Knitting needle	
Glue	Glueing	Glueing paper	
Ice	Icing	Icing sugar	
Need	Needle	Thread the needle	
Yell	Yellow	Yellow paint	
Sew	Sewing	Sewing a dress	

Therapy Targets

CHAPTER 19

THEME: CELEBRATIONS

CONTENTS				
ACTIVITY & PAGE NUMBER	**ACTIVITY**	**CLIENT GROUP**	**LEVEL**	**COMMENTS & SUGGESTIONS**
1(a) Page 258	Celebrations – what do you celebrate?	All	L1–L3	Provide written options for L1.
1(b) Page 259	Celebrations – how do you celebrate?	All	L1–L3	Provide written options for L1.
2(a) Page 260–261	Chinese New Year animals – matching	Language – reading	L2	
2(b) Page 262	Chinese New Year animals – what animal are you?	All	L2–L3	
2(c) Page 263	Chinese New Year animals – anagrams	Language – word recall and spelling	L1–L2	
2(d) Page 264	Chinese New Year animals – naming	Language – word recall and spelling	L2	Provide written names to be matched to the animal for L1.
3 Page 265	Ideas-web: Diwali	All	L2–L3	Provide written answers or pictures for L1 clients.
4 Pages 266–267	Bar & Bat Mitzvah definitions	All	L2–L3	
5(a) Pages 268–269	Ramadan and Eid ul-Fitr – fill in the missing words	All	L2–L3	
5(b) Pages 270–271	Ramadan and Eid ul-Fitr – questions and answers	All	L2–L3	Provide written answers or pictures for L1 clients answer the questions. Ideal as a reading passage.
6 Page 272	Christmas anagrams	Language – spelling and word recall	L2	
7 Page 273	Gifts – discussion	All	L2–L3	
8 Page 274	Weddings word search	Language	L1	

DOI: 10.4324/9781003177852-19

Activity 1(a): Celebrations – what do you celebrate?

Instructions: List five occasions that you celebrate.

1)

2)

3)

4)

5)

Therapy Targets

Activity 1(b): Celebrations – how do you celebrate?

Instructions: Choose a celebration you have listed in Activity 1(a).

Explain how you celebrate this occasion in your family.

TIP: you can speak, write, draw pictures, or mime your answers.

Therapy Targets

Activity 2(a): Chinese New Year animals – matching

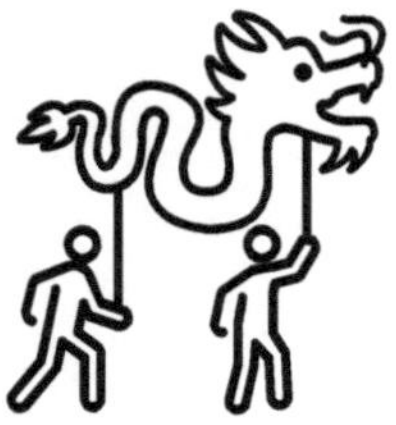

Instructions: Match the attributes to the animal for each of the Chinese years. Answers provided on following page.

Rat	Ox	Tiger	Rabbit	Dragon	Snake
Horse	Goat/sheep	Monkey	Rooster	Dog	Pig

1) Warm, generous, adventurous
2) Hard-working and independent
3) Gentle, affectionate, dislikes arguments
4) Patient, charming, wise
5) Elegant, artistic and good natured
6) Faithful, honest and likes to listen to people's problems
7) Honest, hard-working, loyal
8) Ambitious, clever and imaginative
9) Honest, kind and can be untidy at times
10) Well liked, successful and mischievous
11) Hard-working, confident and organised
12) Confident, hard-working, fun and popular

Therapy Targets

Chinese New Year: Answers to Activity 2(a)

1) Warm, generous, adventurous: Tiger

2) Hard-working and independent: Horse

3) Gentle, affectionate, dislikes arguments: Rabbit

4) Patient, charming, wise: Snake

5) Elegant, artistic and good natured: Goat

6) Faithful, honest and likes to listen to people's problems: Dog

7) Honest, hard-working, loyal: Ox

8) Ambitious, clever and imaginative: Rat

9) Honest, kind and can be untidy at times: Pig

10) Well liked, successful and mischievous: Monkey

11) Hard-working, confident and organised: Rooster

12) Confident, hard-working, fun and popular: Dragon

Activity 2(b): Chinese New Year animals – what animal are you?

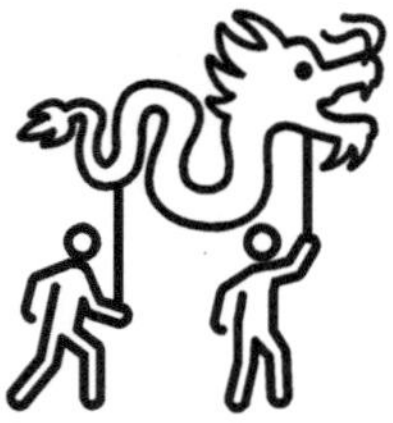

Instructions: Find your Chinese birth year animal.

Rat	Ox	Tiger	Rabbit	Dragon	Snake	Horse	Goat	Monkey	Rooster	Dog	Pig
1900	1901	1902	1903	1904	1905	1906	1907	1908	1909	1910	1911
1912	1913	1914	1915	1916	1917	1918	1919	1920	1921	1922	1923
1924	1925	1926	1927	1928	1929	1930	1931	1932	1933	1934	1935
1936	1937	1938	1939	1940	1941	1942	1943	1944	1945	1946	1947
1948	1949	1950	1951	1952	1953	1954	1955	1956	1957	1958	1959
1960	1961	1962	1963	1964	1965	1966	1967	1968	1969	1970	1971
1972	1973	1974	1975	1976	1977	1978	1979	1980	1981	1982	1983
1984	1985	1986	1987	1988	1989	1990	1991	1992	1993	1994	1995
1996	1997	1998	1999	2000	2001	2002	2003	2004	2005	2006	2007
2008	2009	2010	2011	2012	2013	2014	2015	2016	2017	2018	2019
2020	2021	2022	2023	2024	2025	2026	2027	2028	2029	2030	2031
2032	2033	2034	2035	2036	2037	2038	2039	2040	2041	2042	2043
2044	2045	2046	2047	2048	2049	2050	2051	2052	2053	2054	2055
2056	2057	2058	2059	2060	2061	2062	2063	2064	2065	2066	2067
2068	2069	2070	2071	2072	2073	2074	2075	2076	2077	2078	2079
2080	2081	2082	2083	2084	2085	2086	2087	2088	2089	2090	2091
2092	2093	2094	2095	2096	2097	2098	2099	2100	2101	2102	2103

What year were you born in and what is your Chinese birth year animal?

Can you find the birth year animal for each member of your family?

Therapy Targets

Activity 2(c): Chinese New Year animals – anagrams

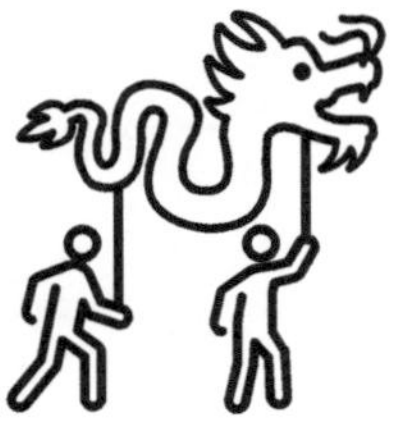

Instructions: Unscramble the letters to name the animals.

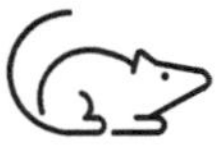	t a r	
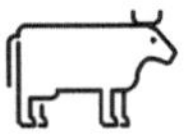	x o	
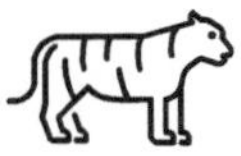	g i e r t	
	b i t b a r	
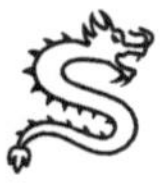	r g n o d a	
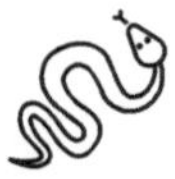	e k n a s	
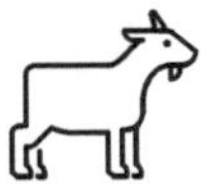	t g a o	
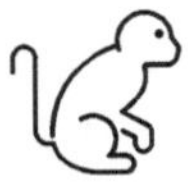	k e m n o y	
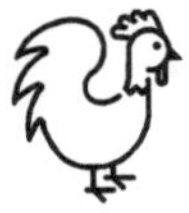	r s o t o r e	
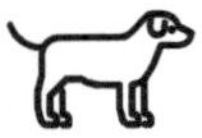	g d o	
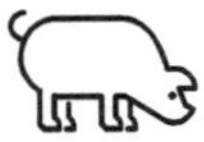	g p i	
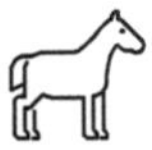	o h s r e	

Therapy Targets

Activity 2(d): Chinese New Year animals – picture naming

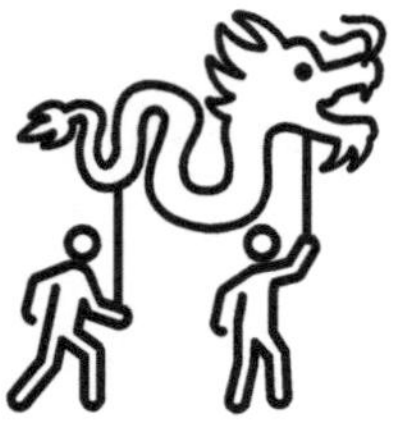

Instructions: Name these animals.

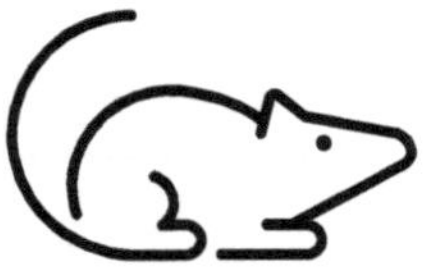

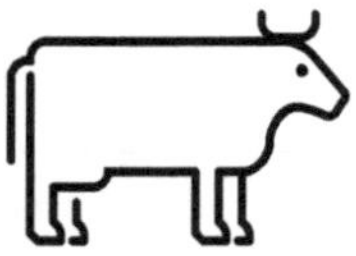

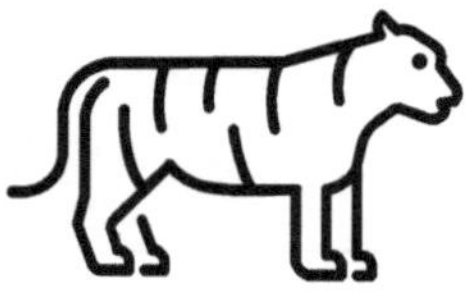

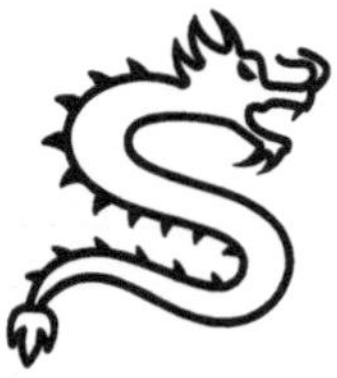

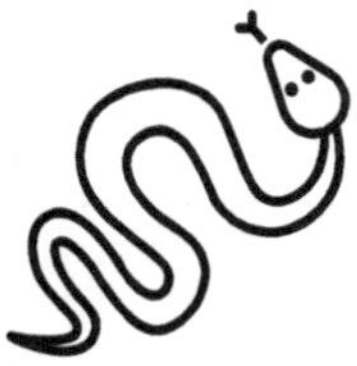

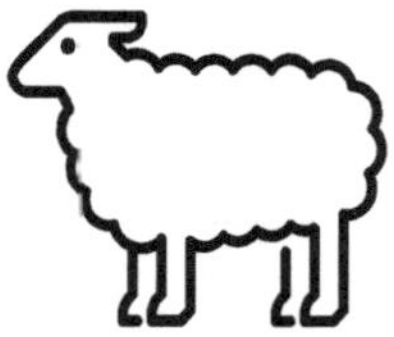

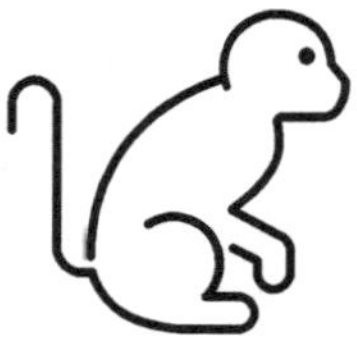

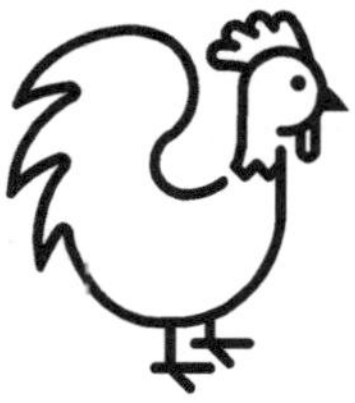

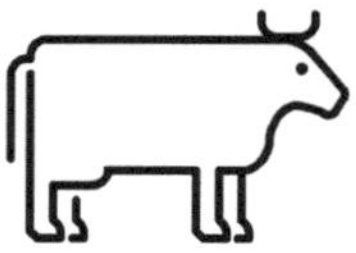

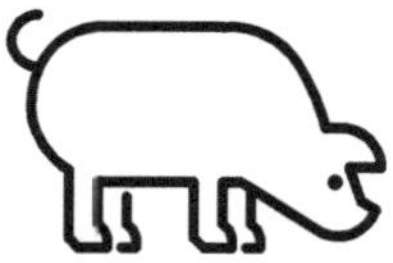

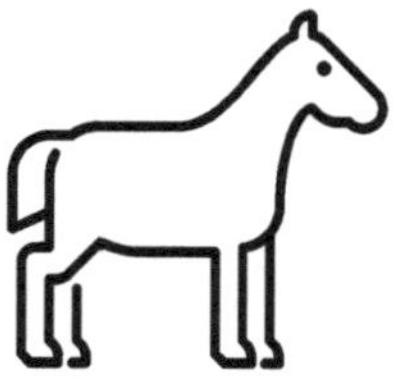

Therapy Targets

Activity 3: Ideas-web: Diwali

Instructions: Answer the questions below about Diwali.

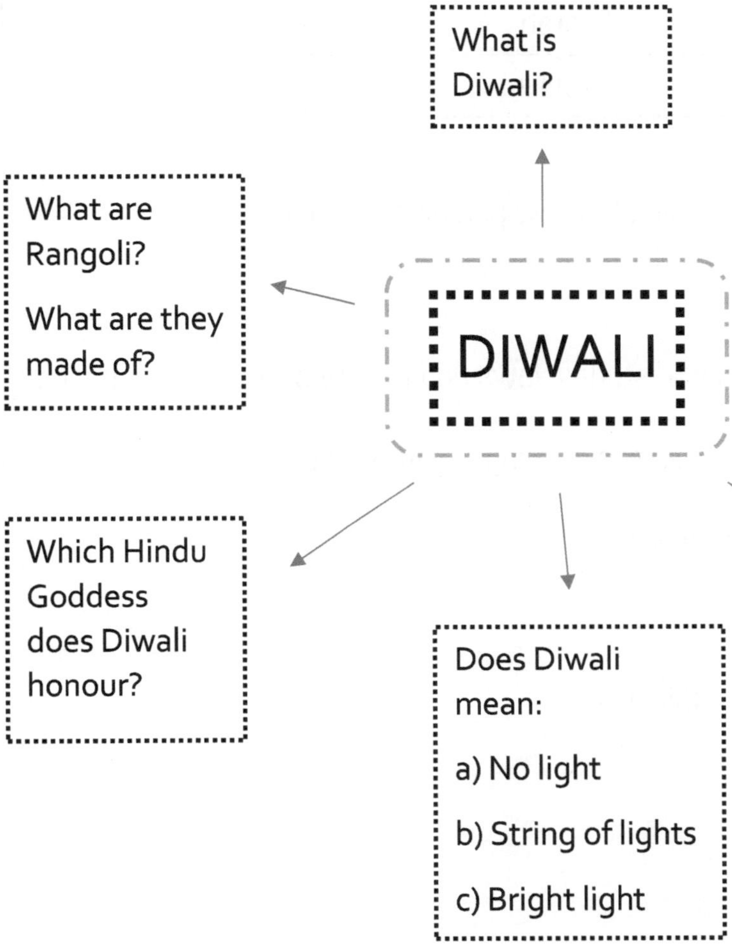

Therapy Targets

Activity 4: Bar Mitzvah; Bat Mitzvah

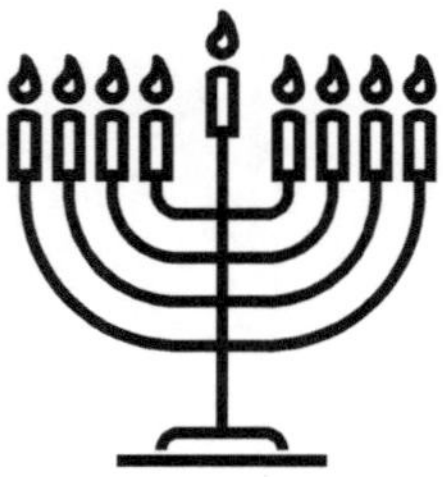

Instructions: Match the word with the description below.

Bar mitzvah	Synagogue	Torah	Rabbi
Bat mitzvah	Minyan	Tefillin	Siddur

1) A pair of black, leather boxes containing Hebrew parchment scrolls:
2) A Jewish prayer book:
3) The Five Books of Moses, the scroll of stories, laws and history of the Jewish people:
4) A group of 10 men over the age of thirteen, coming together to pray:
5) A girl who has reached the age of twelve:
6) The religious teacher:
7) A boy who has reached the age of thirteen:
8) House of worship:

Therapy Targets

Bar Mitzvah; Bat Mitzvah – answers to Activity 4

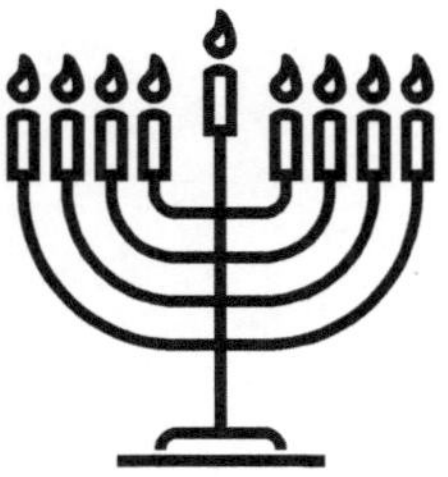

1) A pair of black, leather boxes containing Hebrew parchment scrolls: Tefillin
2) A Jewish prayer book: Siddur
3) The Five Books of Moses, the scroll of stories, laws and history of the Jewish people: Torah
4) A group of 10 men over the age of thirteen, coming together to pray: Minyan
5) A girl who has reached the age of twelve: Bat mitzvah
6) The religious teacher: Rabbi
7) A boy who has reached the age of thirteen: Bar mitzvah
8) House of worship: Synagogue

Extended activity ideas:

a) Swap the activity – provide the explanation and ask the person for the name.

b) Can your client also explain the meanings of these words: Chai (tree of life), Menorah (seven branched candelabra), The Magen David (Star of David).

c) What is Hanukkah – also known as Chanukah? (It commemorates the re-lighting of the Menorah after it had been destroyed by Greek soldiers, recaptured and restored in 139 BCE).

Therapy Targets

Activity 5(a): Ramadan and Eid ul-Fitr

Instructions: Read the passage below and fill in the missing words. Use the words in the box below to help find the right word. Answers provided on the following page.

Ramadan is not a _____________. It is the name of the ninth month of the Islamic _______________. It marks the time when the Qur'an was ______________ as a guide for humankind. Ramadan lasts for one month. During Ramadan, Muslims must _________ between sunrise and sunset. This period is associated with increased devotion through prayer, reading the Qur'an and charity (Zakaat). A traditional greeting during Ramadan is 'Ramadan Mubarak', to which one would _________, 'Ramadan Karim'.

However, the _______ of Ramadan is celebrated with Eid ul-Fitr. This festival lasts for three days. These three days mark the first ____________ days of the Islamic month of Shawwal.

Celebrations for Eid ul-Fitr begin with a prayer at dawn on the first day. Then ___________________ and friends meet up to socialise, eat and exchange gifts, or give to those in need.

Sugary deserts are a large part of the meal. Around the globe, there are many different favourite deserts, depending on the _______________. Eid is time of celebration and goodwill.

families	revealed	end
fast	three	country
celebration	calendar	reply

Therapy Targets

Ramadan and Eid ul-Fitr: Activity 5(a) completed

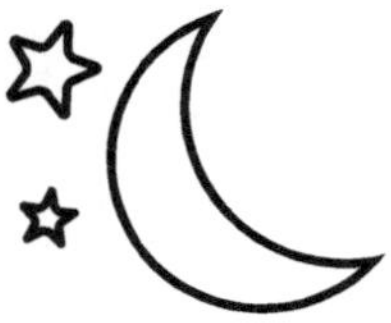

Ramadan is not a celebration. It is the name of the ninth month of the Islamic calendar. It marks the time when the Qur'an was revealed as a guide for humankind. Ramadan lasts for one month. During Ramadan, Muslims must fast between sunrise and sunset. This period is associated with increased devotion through prayer, reading the Qur'an and charity (Zakaat). A traditional greeting during Ramadan is 'Ramadan Mubarak', to which one would reply, 'Ramadan Karim'.

The end of Ramadan is celebrated with Eid ul-Fitr. This festival lasts for three days. These three days mark the first three days of the Islamic month of Shawwal.

Celebrations for Eid ul-Fitr begin with eating dates, then prayers at dawn. Next, family and friends meet up to socialize, eat and exchange gifts. Money is given to those in need.

Sugary desserts are a large part of the meal. Around the globe, there are different favourite deserts, depending on the country. Eid is time of celebration and goodwill.

Activity 5(b): Ramadan and Eid ul-Fitr

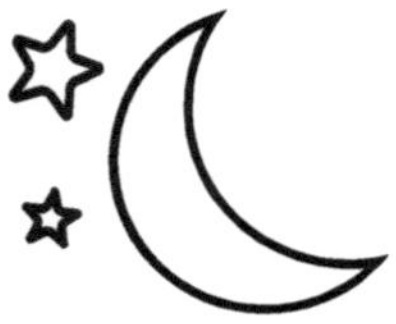

Instructions: Answer the questions below.

1) During Ramadan, are there any exceptions to the rule about not eating and drinking?

2) Why do Muslims fast during Ramadan?

3) What does Eid ul-Fitr mean?

4) What is 'ghusl'?

5) What food is eaten during Eid ul-Fitr?

Therapy Targets

Ramadan and Eid ul-Fitr – answers to Activity 5(b)

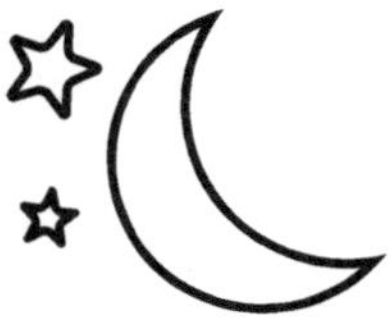

1) During Ramadan, are there any exceptions to the rule about not eating and drinking? *Those who are sick, pregnant, menstruating or are very young.*

2) Why do Muslims fast during Ramadan? *It demonstrates self-discipline, and acts as a reminder of what life is like for others who are not so fortunate.*

3) What does Eid ul-Fitr mean? *Festival of the breaking of the fast.*

4) What is 'ghusl'? *This is a ritual of cleansing the body and dressing in the one's best clothes. It is performed on the first morning of Eid.*

5) What food is eaten during Eid ul-Fitr? *Sweet foods such as dates, date-filled pastries, butter cookies and cakes are frequently eaten. Sweet dishes are also often eaten during the celebrations. Different countries have their own favourites. For example, in Morocco, it might be Laasida and Tagine; in India, Bangladesh and Pakistan, it could be Sheer Khurma.*

Activity 6: Christmas anagrams

Instructions: Complete the phrase – unscramble the letters to find Christmas words.

Jingle ___________ (l l b s e)

Gingerbread ____________ (o h u e s)

Santa ____________ (l a c s u)

Santa's __________ (l v e s e)

Frosty the _________ (n w m a s o n)

The holly and the ___________ (v y i)

Happy ____________ (h r c m s a m i t s)

Wrapping ___________ (p r e p a)

Christmas ____________ (r e t e)

Rudolph the ____________ (d r e n i e e r)

Nativity _____________ (l p y a)

Fairy _____________ (g l i h t s)

25th ______________ (d m c e b r e e)

Therapy Targets

Activity 7: Gifts

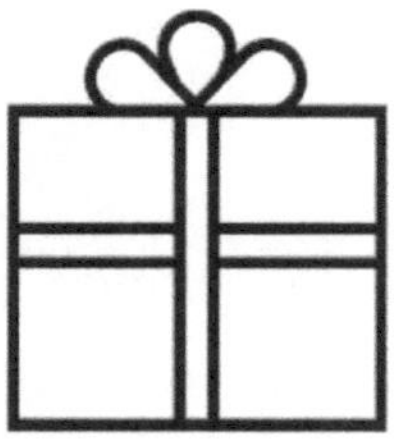

Instructions: Use the questions below to stimulate discussion.

- ❑ What is the best gift you have ever received?
- ❑ What is the worst gift you have ever received?
- ❑ What is the funniest gift you have ever received?
- ❑ Do you think some festivals have become too commercialised?
- ❑ How do you wrap your presents?
- ❑ How could we make gifts more environmentally friendly?

Therapy Targets

Activity 8: Weddings word search

Instructions: Find the wedding words in the letter grid.

music rings groom

bride married vows

G	J	A	R	M	D	B
M	U	S	I	C	E	R
G	D	V	N	B	I	I
V	R	Z	G	L	R	D
O	F	O	S	H	R	E
W	R	T	O	W	A	K
S	U	I	E	M	M	N

Therapy Targets

Activity: Words of increasing length

Instructions: Read across each row. Say the words. Use the words in the third column to make a longer sentence.

The blank boxes at the bottom can be used for your own word sequences.

One syllable	Two syllables	Multisyllabic	Now say a complete sentence using the multisyllabic word or phrase
Birth	Birthday	Happy birthday	
Wrap	Wrapping	Wrapping paper	
Can	Candle	Candlestick	
Light	Lighting	Lighting the candle	
Part	Party	Let's have a party	
Wed	Wedding	Wedding cake	

Therapy Targets

CHAPTER 20

THEME: HEALTH & WELL-BEING

CONTENTS				
ACTIVITY & PAGE NUMBER	**ACTIVITY**	**CLIENT GROUP**	**LEVEL**	**COMMENTS & SUGGESTIONS**
1 Page 278	Word search – a day at the spa	Language	L2–L3	See 'How to use this resource' for ideas on how to extend this activity.
2 Page 279	Word search – relaxing words	Language	L1	
3 Page 280	Healthy drinks – naming task	All	L1–L3	Provide pictures and words for L1 clients to complete this activity.
4 Page 281	Preparing healthy food – sequencing description	All	L2–L3	L1 clients might be able to put into order pre-written sentences.
5 Page 282	Word finder	Language	L1–L3	
6 Page 283	Odd-one-out – relaxation	All	L1–L2	
7 Pages 284–285	Reflexology passage – missing words	All	L3	
8(a) Page 286	Identifying healthy food and drink	Language	L2	
8(b) Page 287	Discussion topics about healthy food and drink	All	L2–L3	Use pictures to facilitate engagement for clients at L1.
9 Page 288	Health and well-being word association	All	L1–L2	Use pictures, mime and written words to facilitate engagement for clients at L1.
10 Page 289	Relaxation practice	All	L1–L3	Simplify the language for L1 clients.

DOI: 10.4324/9781003177852-20

Activity 1: Word search – a day at the spa

Instructions: Find the words below in the letter grid.

yoga	pilates	meditation	relaxation
massage	calm	spa	breathing
pamper	detox	revive	sauna

K	F	R	E	L	A	X	A	T	I	O	N
C	A	A	G	Y	Y	V	D	U	S	E	N
A	Y	P	M	H	O	Z	D	E	T	O	X
L	M	A	S	S	A	G	E	X	I	L	R
M	S	J	U	O	R	S	A	T	K	B	E
F	E	Q	R	E	P	M	A	P	K	W	V
N	T	E	K	E	Y	T	K	N	F	N	I
G	A	T	E	C	I	O	I	L	U	M	V
R	L	S	X	D	P	O	O	L	I	A	E
L	I	T	E	L	O	C	K	E	R	B	S
H	P	M	B	R	E	A	T	H	I	N	G

Therapy Targets

Activity 2: Word search – relaxing words

Instructions: Find the words below in the letter grid.

warm cosy relax calm spa

G	S	P	A	Z	R
W	C	D	X	N	E
A	S	A	R	Y	L
R	B	M	L	O	A
M	F	C	U	M	X
E	C	O	S	Y	I

Therapy Targets

Activity 3: Healthy drinks – naming task

Instructions: Read the sentences below. Write, draw, mime or speak your answers.

1) Name three healthy drinks.

2) Name three drinks to have in moderation.

3) We should have 6–8 healthy drinks a day. How many do you have?

4) What is your favourite drink?

5) What drink is H_2O?

Therapy Targets

Activity 4: Preparing healthy food

Instructions: Describe how to make the following:

1) smoothie

2) salad

3) stir fry

4) fruit salad

5) fish pie

Therapy Targets

Activity 5: Finding smaller words in a longer word

Instructions: How many little words can you find in the word meditation? They do not have to be words related to the word meditation.

MEDITATION

Extended activity ideas:

- ❑ Make a sentence with the words you find.
- ❑ What does meditation mean?
- ❑ Do you meditate or practise relaxation?
    - ❑ Explain what you do?
    - ❑ How does it help you?

Therapy Targets

Activity 6: Odd-one-out – relaxation

Instructions: Identify the odd-one-out in each row.

Relaxing	Sky-diving	Meditating	Breathing
Whirlpool	Sauna	Canal	Hot-tub
Fighting	Breathing	Laughing	Sleeping
Reflexology	Aromatherapy	Reiki	Surgery
Yoga	Pilates	Wrestling	Swimming
Facial	Dental-filling	Manicure	Pedicure
Petrol	Lavender	Jasmine	Chamomile

Therapy Targets

Activity 7(a): Reflexology passage

Instructions: Read this passage. Use the words in the box to fill in the missing spaces.

body	years	feet	century	Egyptians	reflexology

Reflexology is a non-medical treatment that dates back to the ancient _______. It involves applying pressure to the feet to promote the natural healing of the body.

Pressure is applied to specific areas on the ______ that represent the different areas of the body.

Through the ages, different civilizations have developed the concept of different parts of the foot representing different parts of the _____. For example, roughly 3000 ______ ago in China, a medical paper was written called, 'Tao of Foot Centre'. This text explained how the foot was related to the rest of the body.

In the 21st __________ the Russians explored how the nerves on the surface of the skin were linked to the internal organs of the body. They discovered that the organs could be altered by external reflexes. This understanding of how the systems worked progressed, and in 1917 the term _____________ was coined by the Russians.

Therapy Targets

Activity 7(b): Reflexology passage – complete passage

Instructions: See 'how to use this resource' chapter for ideas on how to use the completed passage.

Reflexology is a non-medical treatment that dates back to the ancient Egyptians. It involves applying pressure to the feet to promote the natural healing of the body.

Pressure is applied to specific areas on the feet that represent the different areas of the body.

Through the ages, different civilizations have developed the concept of different parts of the foot representing different parts of the body. For example, roughly 3000 years ago in China, a medical paper was written called, 'Tao of Foot Centre'. This text explained how the foot was related to the rest of the body.

In the 21st century the Russians explored how the nerves on the surface of the skin were linked to the internal organs of the body. They discovered that the organs could be altered by external reflexes. This understanding of how the systems worked progressed, and in 1917 the term 'reflexology' was coined by the Russians.

Therapy Targets

Activity 8(a): Healthy food and drink

Instructions: Identify which foods below might be considered healthy.

chocolate	oats	carrots	chips
nuts	avocado	okra	oil
cumin	ghee	beer	salt
raisins	seeds	rice	turmeric
wine	sage	burgers	figs
garlic	dates	milk	butter
water	onions	thyme	crisps
lychees	cola	banana	pasta
cheese	gin	yam	cream

Therapy Targets

Activity 8(b): Healthy food and drink

Instructions: Using the table on the previous page, discuss the questions below.

a) Which of these foods and drinks do you like the most?

b) Which of these foods do you avoid or dislike?

c) Should you avoid all unhealthy food and drink?

d) Explain the saying:

"A little of what you fancy does you good"

e) Can you explain what different nutrients we get from some of the food in the table above.

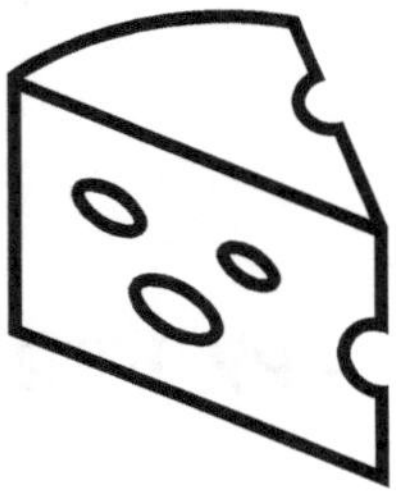

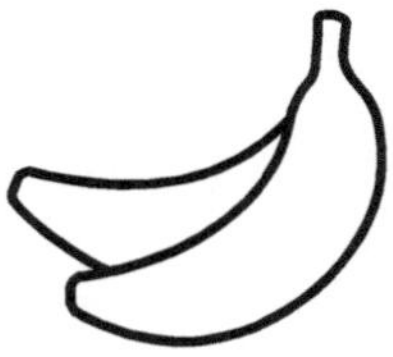

Therapy Targets

Activity 9: Health and well-being

Instructions: What words do you associate with health and well-being?

HEALTH AND WELL-BEING

Therapy Targets

Activity 10: Relaxation practice

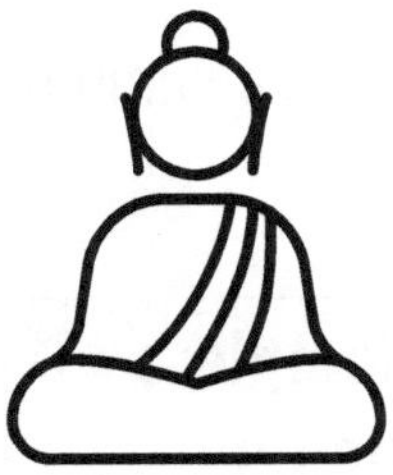

Instructions: Read this passage to your client to help them relax.

Alternatively, use the passage as a language exercise (see 'How to use this resource' at the beginning of the book).

Take a deep breath and breath out. Now take a deep breath and hold it for a couple of seconds, breathe out. Close your eyes and breathe in for a count of three, breathe out for a count of five; pause and breathe in and out like this for a few moments.

Imagine you are sitting by a calm lake. It is a warm day with a pleasant breeze. You are on a soft blanket, and you decide to lie down. Listen to the sounds around you. Perhaps you can hear birds singing or the sound of the light wind in the trees.

You can feel the warmth of the sun on your body, relaxing it. The gentle breeze drifts over you, blowing the tension away. As you smell the sweet scent of the flowers, you feel yourself drifting and letting go.

Rest quietly for a few moments. Enjoy the peace and calm.

When you are ready, begin to wriggle your toes and fingers; become aware of your surroundings. Take a deep breath and as you breathe out, open your eyes.

Take this feeling of calm with you for the rest of your day.

Therapy Targets

Activity: Words of increasing length

Instructions: Read across each row. Say the words. Use the words in the third column to make a longer sentence.

One syllable	Two syllables	Multisyllabic	Now say a complete sentence using the multisyllabic word or phrase
Mind	Mindful	Mindfulness	
Health	Healthy	Healthy living	
Pool	Whirlpool	Relaxing whirlpool	
Soothe	Soothing	Soothing treatment	
Calm	Calming	Calming music	
Mass	Massage	Massaging	

Therapy Targets

APPENDIX 1-BLANK TEMPLATES

ACROSTIC

Instructions:

Can you find words that begin with each letter of the word …………………………………..

Try to make the words you find relevant to the topic of …………………………………………

If you are feeling brave you might want to write a poem.

Therapist:

Example: DOG

D – dutiful

O – obedient

G – good dog!

BOARD GAME 1

FINISH	47	46	45	44	43
37	38	39	40	41	42
36	35	34	33	32	31
25	26	27	28	29	30
24	23	22	21	20	19
13	14	15	16	17	18
12	11	10	9	8	7
1 START	2	3	4	5	6

BOARD GAME 2

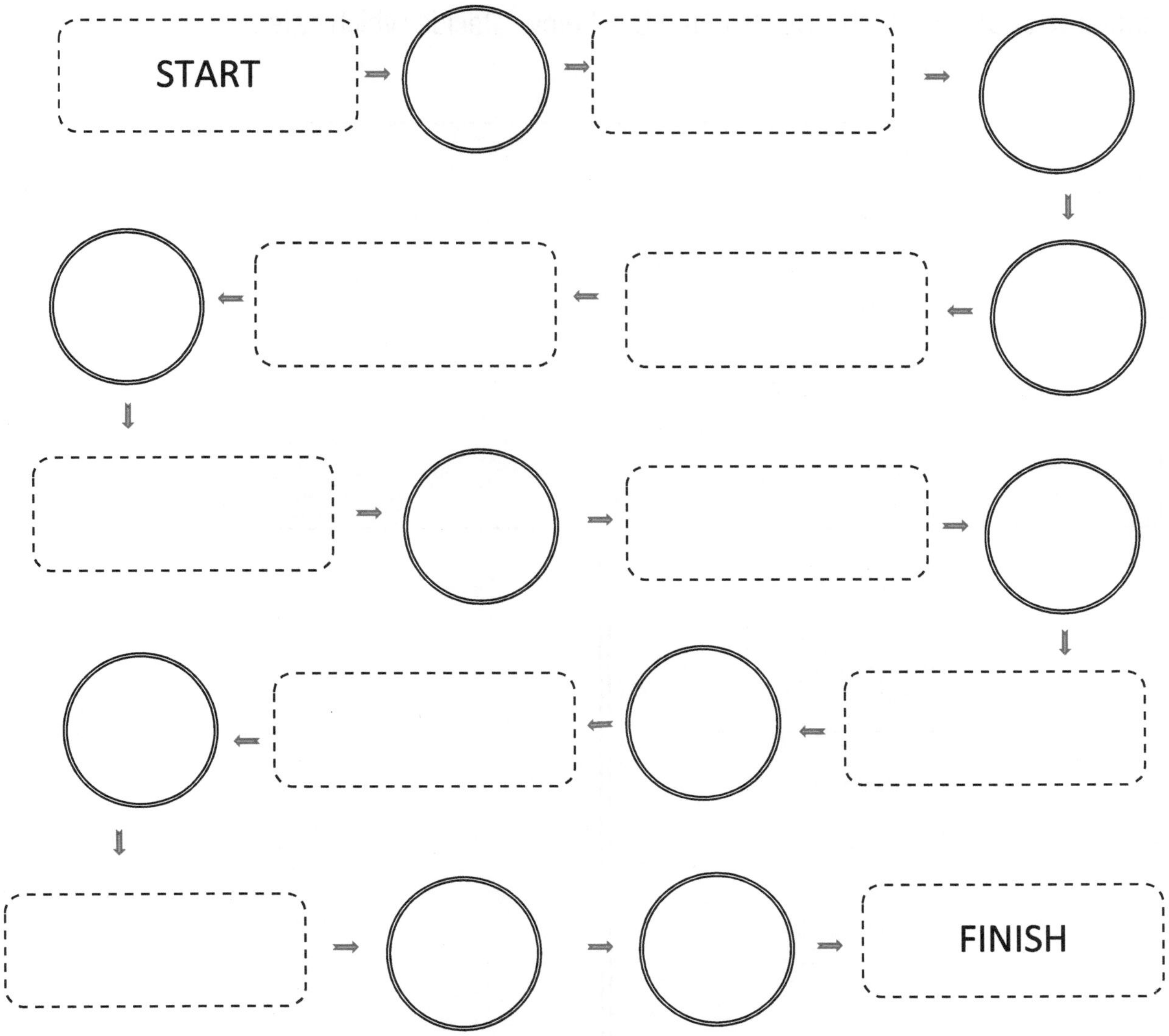

Activity: Categorising objects or actions.

Instructions: Look at the words in the box below. Decide which category they belong to.

CROSSWORD

PEN & PAPER GRID-WARS

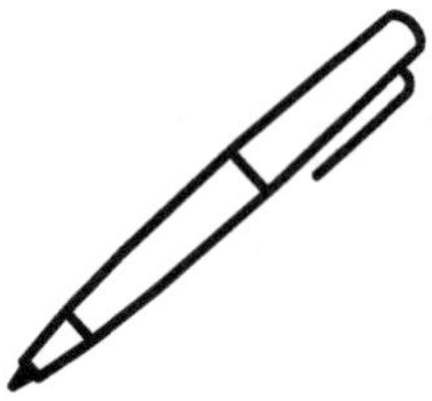

Instructions:

Decide on the items to be found (e.g. weeds, balls etc).

Each player marks their grid without showing the other person.

Take it in turns to find the other person's objects by giving a grid reference, for example: G 4

Who can find the most items?

H								
G								
F								
E								
D								
C								
B								
A								
	1	2	3	4	5	6	7	8

WORD SEARCH

Find the words below in the letter grid

Words of increasing length

Instructions: Read across each row. Say the words.

Use the words in the third column to make your own sentence.

One syllable	Two syllables	Multisyllabic	Now say a complete sentence using the multisyllabic word or phrase

Activity: Making sentences

Therapist instructions: Complete the boxes below, organising them into different categories (e.g. noun, verb, adjective, adverb).

Client instructions: Choose one word from each category. Put the words together to make a sentence.

Category one

Category two

Category three

Do the sentences make sense?

Can you write three more of your own using the words in the boxes?

Can you write three more sentences using your own words?

Activity: Making sentences

Therapist instructions: Complete the boxes below, organising them into the different categories (e.g. conjunctions, adjectives, adverbs and prepositions).

Client instructions: Choose one word from each category. Put the words together to make a sentence.

Category one

Category two

Category three

Category four

Category five

Activity: Making sentences

Therapist instructions: Complete the boxes below, organising them into the different categories (e.g. noun, verb, adjective, adverb).

Client instructions: Roll a dice. Select a card from each category that corresponds with the number on your dice.

(You could use the same number for each category, or roll the dice three times for a different number for each category.)

Use the selected words to create a sentence.

Category one (e.g. noun, adjective)

1	4
2	5
3	6

Category two (e.g. verb, conjunction)

1	4
2	5
3	6

Category three (e.g. adverb, determiner)

1	4
2	5
3	6

Do the sentences make sense?

Can you write three more of your own using the words in the boxes?

Can you write three more sentences using your own words?

APPENDIX 2-ABOUT ME QUESTIONNAIRE

To make therapy more relevant, please tell me a little bit about yourself.

Please have a look at the questions below and provide as much information as you want.

If there are any questions you would rather not complete, leave them blank.

This information will remain confidential.

My name:
I like to be called:

Where I was born:
Where I went to school, college or university:
Jobs I have had:
My family:
My friends:

My pets and their names:

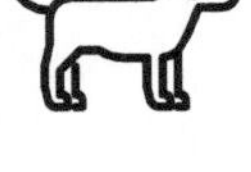

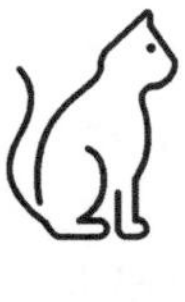

My hobbies and interests are:

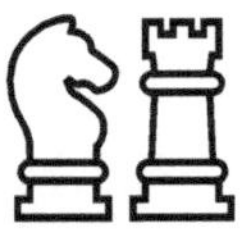

Sport

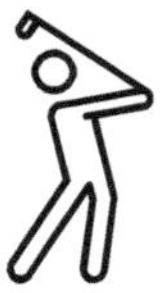

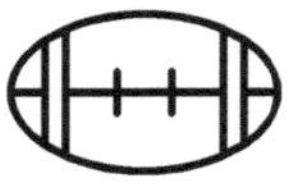

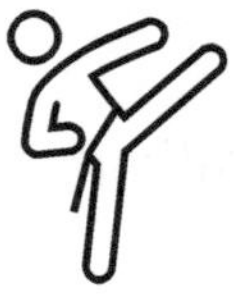

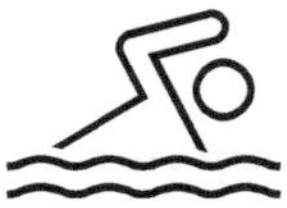

I like to watch:

I like to play:

Music

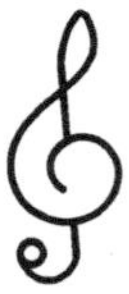

I like listening to:

I play an instrument:

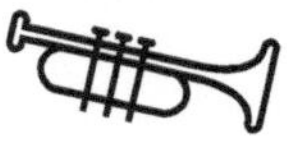

Favourite films, TV and radio programmes:

Using a mobile phone, computer, iPad or tablet:
(circle any that apply)
I am confident enough to use these:
Frequently *Sometimes* *Never*

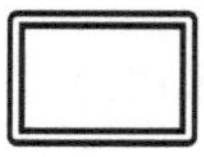

I use / would like to use my phone, tablet or computer for:
(e.g. shopping, games, video calls)

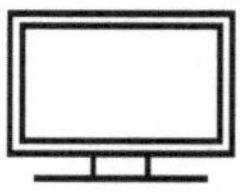

I like to read:
Novels
Biographies / autobiographies / eBooks? (Kindle)
Information books (state which topic):
Magazines (which ones?)
Newspapers (which ones?)
Poetry
Emails
Other (please specify)

I need or want to write:
Letters or cards:
Shopping lists:
Phone numbers:
Notes:
Complex information such as minutes of meetings/lecture notes:
Texts:
Emails:
Other (please specify):

Other information you might like to know about me:

BIBLIOGRAPHY

Note: Not every reference in this Bibliography is directly cited in the text but has been left in for the reader's interest.

American Speech-Language-Hearing Association (n.d.). *Fluency Disorders* [online]. Available at: https://www.asha.org/practice-portal/clinical-topics/fluency-disorders/#collapse_6 [Accessed 2021].

Andrea, M., Andrea, M. and Figueira, M.L. (2018). Self-perception of quality of life in patients with functional voice disorders: The effects of psychological and vocal acoustic variables. *European Archives of Oto-Rhino-Laryngology*, 275(11), pp.2745–2754.

Arkin, S. and Mahendra, N. (2001). Discourse analysis of Alzheimer's patients before and after intervention: Methodology and outcomes. *Aphasiology*, 15(6), pp.533–569.

Balchin, R., Hersh, D., Grantis, J. and Godfrey, M. (2020). "Ode to confidence": Poetry groups for dysarthria in multiple sclerosis. *International Journal of Speech-Language Pathology*, 22(3), pp.347–358.

Bannink, F. (2010). *1001 solution-focused questions – handbook for solution-focused interviewing*. 2nd ed. [online]. W.W. Norton & Co, p.229. Available at: https://www.booktopia.com.au/1001-solution-focused-questions-fredrike-bannink/book/9780393706345.html.

Best, W., Greenwood, A., Grassly, J., Herbert, R., Hickin, J. and Howard, D. (2013). Aphasia rehabilitation: Does generalisation from anomia therapy occur and is it predictable? A case series study. *Cortex*, 49(9), pp.2345–2357.

Blomgren, M. and Goberman, A.M. (2008). Revisiting speech rate and utterance length manipulations in stuttering speakers. *Journal of Communication Disorders*, 41(2), pp.159–178.

Bruce, C. and Newton, C. (2018). "What's cooking?" A comparison of an activity-oriented and a table-top programme of therapy on the language performance of people with aphasia. *International Journal of Language & Communication Disorders*, 54(3), pp.430–443.

Cardell, E. and Lawrie, M. (2013). *Semantic and naming therapy: An integrated approach: linking the semantic system and the lexicons*. Milton Keynes: Speechmark Publishing Ltd.

Carragher, M., Conroy, P., Sage, K. and Wilkinson, R. (2012). Can impairment-focused therapy change the everyday conversations of people with aphasia? A review of the literature and future directions. *Aphasiology*, 26(7), pp.895–916.

Cooney, A. and O'Shea, E. (2018). The impact of life story work on person-centred care for people with dementia living in long-stay care settings in Ireland. *Dementia*, 18(7–8), pp.2731–2746. Online first.

Dromey, C. and Shim, E. (2008). The effects of divided attention on speech motor, verbal fluency, and manual task performance. *Journal of Speech, Language, and Hearing Research*, 51(5), pp.1171–1182.

Dromey, C., Jarvis, E., Sondrup, S., Nissen, S., Foreman, K.B. and Dibble, L.E. (2010). Bidirectional interference between speech and postural stability in individuals with Parkinson's disease. International Journal of Speech-Language Pathology [online], 12(5), pp.446–454. Available at: https://scholarsarchive.byu.edu/cgi/viewcontent.cgi?article=2810&context=facpub [Accessed 11 Nov. 2020].

Elman, R.J. (2007). *Group treatment of neurogenic communication disorders: The expert clinician's approach*. San Diego, CA: Plural Pub.

Elman, R.J. and Bernstein-Ellis, E. (1999). The efficacy of group communication treatment in adults with chronic aphasia. *Journal of Speech, Language, and Hearing Research*, 42(2), pp.411–419.
Enderby, P. (2013). Disorders of communication: Dysarthria. In: *Handbook of clinical neurology*. Elsevier.
Enderby, P.M. and Enderby, J.A. (2015). *Therapy outcome measures for rehabilitation professionals*. Guildford: J&R Press, Cop.
Fujii, S. and Wan, C.Y. (2014). The role of rhythm in speech and language rehabilitation: The SEP hypothesis. *Frontiers in Human Neuroscience*, 8.
Herbert, R., Best, W., Hickin, J., Howard, D. and Osborne, F. (2001). Phonological and orthographic approaches to the treatment of word retrieval in aphasia. *International Journal of Language & Communication Disorders*, 36(s1) Supplement, pp.7–12.
Herbert, R., Best, W., Hickin, J., Howard, D. and Osborne, F. (2003). Combining lexical and interactional approaches to therapy for word finding deficits in aphasia. *Aphasiology*, 17(12), pp.1163–1186.
Herbert, R., Gregory, E. and Best, W. (2013). Syntactic versus lexical therapy for anomia in acquired aphasia: Differential effects on narrative and conversation. *International Journal of Language & Communication Disorders*, 49(2), pp.162–173.
Hilari, K. and Northcott, S. (2017). "Struggling to stay connected": Comparing the social relationships of healthy older people and people with stroke and aphasia. *Aphasiology*, 31(6), pp.674–687.
Holmes, R. ed. (1980). *A country calendar of rural rhymes*. London: Eyre Methuen, p.52.
Huber, J.E. and Darling, M. (2011). Effect of Parkinson's Disease on the production of structured and unstructured speaking tasks: Respiratory physiologic and linguistic considerations. *Journal of Speech, Language, and Hearing Research*, 54(1), pp.33–46.
Jordan, L. and Bryan, K. (2001). Seeing the Person? Disability Theories and Speech and Language Therapy. *International Journal of Language & Communication Disorders*, 36(s1) Supplement, pp.453–458.
Kiresuk, T.J. and Sherman, R.E. (1968). Goal attainment scaling: A general method for evaluating comprehensive community mental health programs. Community Mental Health Journal, [online] 4(6), pp.443–453. Available at: https://link.springer.com/article/10.1007%2FBF01530764 [Accessed 24 Sep. 2021].
Kitwood, T. (2011). The person comes first: Dementia reconsidered. In: *Adult lives: A life course perspective*. Policy Press.
Lock, S., Wilkinson, R., Bryan, K. and Bruce, C. (2008). *SPPARC: Supporting partners of people with aphasia in relationships and conversation*. Milton Keynes: Speechmark.
Lucey, J., Evans, D. and Maxfield, N.D. (2019). Temperament in adults who stutter and its association with stuttering frequency and quality-of-life impacts. *Journal of Speech, Language, and Hearing Research*, 62(8), pp.2691–2702.
Martin, S. and Lockhart, M. (2013). *Working with voice disorders*. Milton Keynes: Speechmark.
Misono, S., Meredith, L., Peterson, C.B. and Frazier, P.A. (2016). New perspective on psychosocial distress in patients with dysphonia: The moderating role of perceived control. *Journal of Voice*, 30(2), pp.172–176.
NICE (2018). *Overview | Dementia: Assessment, management and support for people living with dementia and their carers | Guidance | NICE*. [online] Nice.org.uk. Available at: https://www.nice.org.uk/guidance/ng97.
Parker, V. ed. (2000). *100 great poems: Favourite poems and their poets*. Essex: Miles Kelly, pp.46–47.
Patterson, J.P. (2001). The effectiveness of cueing hierarchies as a treatment for word retrieval impairment. *Perspectives on Neurophysiology and Neurogenic Speech and Language Disorders*, 11(2), p.11.
Pietro, M.J.S. and Boczko, F. (1998). The Breakfast Club: Results of a study examining the effectiveness of a multi-modality group communication treatment. *American Journal of Alzheimer's Disease*, 13(3), pp.146–158.
Ramig, L. and Fox, C. (2008) LSVT LOUD Training and Certification Workshop. GleeCo, LSVT Global, LLC.
Royal College of Speech and Language Therapists (RCSLT) (n.d.). Stroke fact sheet. [online] Available at: https://www.rcslt.org/wp-content/uploads/2021/09/rcslt-stroke-factsheet.pdf

Sanot-Pietro, M.J. and Ostuni, E. (2003). *Successful communication with persons with Alzheimer's disease: An in-service manual*. St. Louis, MO.: Butterworth-Heinemann.

Scholl, D.I., McCabe, P., Nickels, L. and Ballard, K.J. (2021). Outcomes of semantic feature analysis treatment for aphasia with and without apraxia of speech. *International Journal of Language & Communication Disorders*, 56(3), pp.485–500.

Walshe, M. and Miller, N. (2011). Living with acquired dysarthria: The speaker's perspective. *Disability and Rehabilitation*, 33(3), pp.195–203.

Währborg, P. (1991). *Assessment & management of emotional reactions to brain damage & aphasia*. Kibworth, Leics.: Far Communications.

Whillans, C., Lawrie, M., Cardell, E.A., Kelly, C. and Wenke, R. (2020). A systematic review of group intervention for acquired dysarthria in adults. *Disability and Rehabilitation*, pp.1–17.

World Health Organization (2001). *International Classification of Functioning, Disability and Health (ICF)*. [online] www.who.int. Available at: https://www.who.int/standards/classifications/international-classification-of-functioning-disability-and-health.

www.kcl.ac.uk (n.d.). King's College London – *GAS – Goal Attainment Scaling in rehabilitation*. [online] Available at: https://www.kcl.ac.uk/cicelysaunders/resources/tools/gas.

Yaruss, J.S. (2010). Assessing quality of life in stuttering treatment outcomes research. *Journal of Fluency Disorders*, 35(3), pp.190–202.